CRASH COURSE
Rheumatology and Orthopaedics

FIRST EDITION

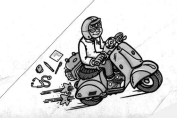

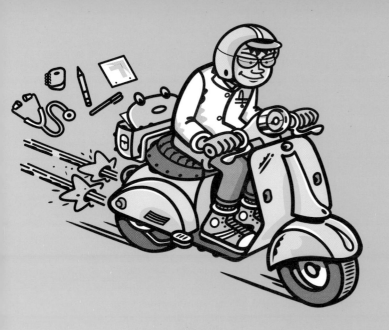

Series editor
Daniel Horton-Szar
BSc (Hons), MB BS (Hons)
Northgate Medical Practice
Canterbury
Kent

Faculty advisors
Michael Snaith
MD, FRCP
Senior Clinical Lecturer in
Rheumatology
University of Sheffield
Honorary Consultant Rheumatologist
Royal Hallamshire Hospital
Sheffield

Andrew Hamer
MB, ChB, MD, FRCS (Orth)
Consultant Orthopaedic Surgeon
Northern General Hospital
Sheffield

Rheumatology and Orthopaedics

FIRST EDITION

Annabel Coote

MBChB, MRCP
Specialist Registrar in Rheumatology
Royal Hallamshire Hospital
Sheffield

Paul Haslam

MBChB, FRCS Ed, FRCS (Tr & Orth)
Specialist Registrar in Orthopaedics
Northern General Hospital
Sheffield

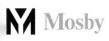 Mosby

Edinburgh • London • New York • Oxford • Philadelphia • St Louis • Sydney • Toronto 2004

MOSBY
An imprint of Elsevier Limited

Commissioning Editor	Fiona Conn
Project Development Manager	Fiona Conn
Project Manager	Frances Affleck
Designer	Andy Chapman
Illustration Management	Bruce Hogarth

First published 2004
 Reprinted 2007

ISBN 978 0 7234 3350 7

British Library Cataloguing in Publication Data
A catalogue record for this book is available from the British Library

Library of Congress Cataloging in Publication Data
A catalog record for this book is available from the Library of Congress

Note
Medical knowledge is constantly changing. Standard safety precautions must be followed, but as new research and clinical experience broaden our knowledge, changes in treatment and drug therapy may become necessary or appropriate. Readers are advised to check the most current product information provided by the manufacturer of each drug to be administered to verify the recommended dose, the method and duration of administration, and contraindications. It is the responsibility of the practitioner, relying on experience and knowledge of the patient, to determine dosages and the best treatment for each individual patient. Neither the Publisher nor the authors assume any liability for any injury and/or damage to persons or property arising from this publication.

The Publisher

Working together to grow
libraries in developing countries

www.elsevier.com | www.bookaid.org | www.sabre.org

ELSEVIER   BOOK AID
             International   Sabre Foundation

ELSEVIER   your source for books,
            journals and multimedia
            in the health sciences
www.elsevierhealth.com

The
Publisher's
policy is to use
**paper manufactured
from sustainable forests**

Typeset by Kolam, Pondicherry, India
Printed in China

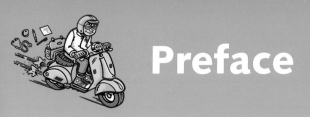

Preface

Over the last six years since the first editions of *Crash Course* were published, there have been many changes in medicine, and in the way it is taught. The second editions have been largely rewritten to take these changes into account, and keep *Crash Course* up to date for the twenty-first century. New material has been added to include recent research and all pharmacological and disease management information has been updated in line with current best practice. We've listened to feedback from hundreds of medical students who have been using *Crash Course* and have improved the structure and layout of the books accordingly: pathology and disease management material has been moved closer to the diagnostic skills chapters; there are more MCQs and now we have Extended Matching Questions as well, with explanations of each answer. We have also included 'Further Reading' sections where appropriate to highlight important papers and studies that you should be aware of, and the clarity of text and figures is better than ever. We are also extending the range of the series with this, and other new titles that follow the same successful *Crash Course* formula.

The principles on which we developed the series remain the same, however. Clinical medicine is a huge subject, and teaching on the wards can sometimes be sporadic because of the competing demands of patient care. The last thing a student needs when finals are approaching is to waste time assembling information from different sources, or wading through pages of irrelevant detail. As before, *Crash Course* brings you all the information you need in compact, manageable volumes that integrate an approach to common patient presentations with clinical skills, pathology and management of the relevant diseases. We still tread the fine line between producing clear, concise text and providing enough detail for those aiming at distinction. The series is still written by junior doctors with recent exam experience, in partnership with senior faculty members from across the UK.

I wish you the best of luck in your future careers!

Dr Dan Horton-Szar
Series Editor

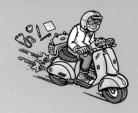

Author Preface

Most people, at some time, will suffer from a musculoskeletal problem, ranging from a sprained ankle or back ache to a broken leg or arthritis.

As a medical student going home for Christmas you will be asked for an opinion on your mate's injured knee, your auntie's bunions and your father's sciatica. (All these scenarios happened to us!) We hope this book prepares you for these embarrassing situations!

It has been estimated that musculoskeletal symptoms are responsible for one in four GP consultations. We can guarantee that, no matter what medical or surgical specialty you choose to practise, you will be exposed to patients with aches and pains in their bones and joints.

Whilst primarily aimed at medical students this book would also be of use to doctors in training, physiotherapists, occupational therapists and nurses.

We hope that you enjoy the book, pass your exams, get drunk and then follow a career in orthopaedics or rheumatology.

Annabel Coote
Paul Haslam

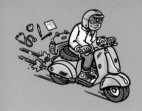

Acknowledgements

To the senior authors AJH and MLS and Dr RS Amos for his assistance with the chapter on Paediatric joint disease.

AC

The senior authors AJH and MS.

Dr Moore consultant radiologist Northern General Hospital Sheffield for the loan of his x-ray collection.

Dr Highland (Ade) SpR radiology Northern General Hospital Sheffield for his advice and help with the investigations chapter.

Dr A Rash (Uma) SpR Medicine Northern General Hospital Sheffield for his help with osteoporosis and spelling.

Ryan for breaking his tibia.

PH

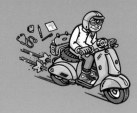

Dedication

To family and friends for their patience and support during the production of this book.

AC

For Mum and Dad, Andrey and Freddie, and Nan.

PH

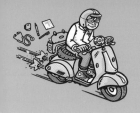

Contents

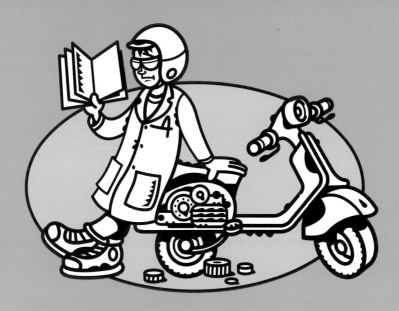

THE PATIENT PRESENTS WITH

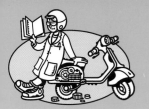

1. Regional Pain

Back, hip and leg pain

One of the most common presentations to a GP is that of back, hip and/or leg pain. 80% of the population will have an episode of back pain at some time in their lives.

The patient may have one or any combination of the three symptoms. An important point to note is that many patients do not know where the hip joint is and most will point to the iliac crest or further posteriorly towards the sacroiliac joint and tell you this is their hip! Other misconceptions abound: one patient may tell you his sciatica is playing up or another that her slipped disc has 'popped out again'.

So when faced with such a patient the physician must decide, on the basis of the history and examination, whether the pain is from the back or the hip joint and if what the patient is telling you is correct!

Differential diagnosis
- Simple low back pain (see Ch. 21).
- Osteoarthritis (see Ch. 8).
  —Hip
  —Spine
- Prolapsed intervertebral disc (see Ch. 21).
- Rheumatoid or other inflammatory arthritis (see Chs 9 and 10).
- Vertebral crush fracture (see Ch. 12).
- Avascular necrosis of hip.
- Spinal stenosis/spondylolisthesis (see Ch. 21).
- Malignancy (see Ch. 20).
- Discitis (see Ch. 21).
- Abdominal causes (referred, e.g. pancreatitis/dissecting aortic aneurysm).

History focusing on back, hip and leg pain
There are essentially four different presentations (Fig. 1.1):
- Back pain.
- Back and leg pain.
- Hip pain ± leg pain.
- Leg pain.

Back pain
Simple low back pain
Acute low back pain without radiation into the leg suggests simple low back pain—particularly if the

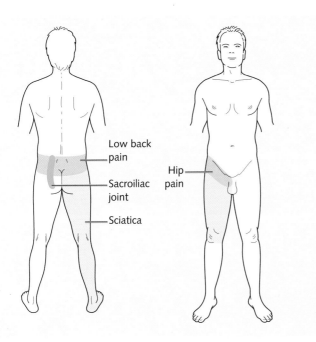

Fig. 1.1 Patterns of pain around the back, leg and hip.

Low back pain

Sacroiliac joint

Sciatica

Hip pain

patient gives a history of lifting or straining, and the pain is worse on movement and activity (so-called 'mechanical pain'). The pain is usually described as a band across the back and may be extremely severe.

Signs of sinister back pain
If the pain is unrelenting, chronic and non-mechanical in nature—particularly in the elderly—a malignant cause such as spinal metastases must be excluded. Night pain is a feature of sinister back pain. If the patient also has a fever and is generally unwell discitis must be considered.

Pain that originates in the abdomen and radiates into the back may well be abdominal.

 Serious emergencies like a ruptured abdominal aortic aneurysm can present with back pain.

Back and leg pain
Back and leg pain suggests that there is nerve root entrapment.

Sciatica
True sciatica radiates down the back of the leg and into the foot. It may be of acute onset from a specific incident, and is typically constant with acute exacerbations lasting seconds. The nature of the pain is like an electric shock and can be very severe. It is aggravated in certain positions such as standing straight and by sneezing or coughing and relieved by bending forward with the knee flexed. Over time the pain usually settles.

Spinal stenosis
In spinal stenosis the patient typically has back pain, and the leg pain comes on after walking and is relieved by rest, so called spinal claudication.

Facet joint osteoarthritis
Facet joint osteoarthritis of the spine can also radiate into the leg but the pain does not extend below the knee and is aching in character.

Hip pain ± leg pain
True hip joint pain is felt in the groin and can radiate down the front of the thigh to the knee. The pain of an arthritic hip is of gradual onset deep, gnawing pain and can be unrelenting. Night pain may be present.

A fractured hip is a common emergency presentation in elderly patients. Usually there is a clear history of a fall but this is not always the case, particularly in confused patients.

Leg pain
Occasionally a prolapsed intervertebral disc presents with leg pain only (sciatica) without the back pain.

Loss of function/degree of disability
Patients will complain of limitation of certain activities, which may be recreational, work related or more basic activities of daily living.

It is important to know how much impact the disorder has on normal day-to-day living.

Back pain is the leading cause of sickness from work.

Associated symptoms
It is essential to ask about urinary or bowel disturbance in any patient with back pain. Incontinence of urine or faeces suggests a cauda equina syndrome needing prompt investigation and treatment.

Numbness, pins and needles and weakness of the foot should be elicited in the history and suggest true sciatica.

Weight loss and a history of previous malignancy indicate possible malignancy.

 Patients can present 'off their legs' and occasionally this is due to malignancy and spinal cord compression.

Examination focusing on back, hip and leg pain
General examination
Look at the patient: weight loss, anaemia and general ill-health may suggest malignancy.

Look at the posture and gait:
- A stooped posture with flexion of the knee suggests sciatica.
- A frail old lady with a stooped posture may have osteoporotic fractures.
- A very stiff spine may be simple low back pain or ankylosing spondylitis.

- Fixed flexion of the hip with an antalgic or Trendelenburg gait is likely to be hip pathology. There may be a limb length discrepancy.
- Look for deformity of the spine, previous scars, wasting and any lower limb deformity.

Perform the Trendelenburg and Thomas tests as described in Chapter 27. These are tests aimed at examining the hip and if positive suggest hip pathology.

Palpation
- With the patient standing, palpate the spine and surrounding muscles for tenderness. In simple low back pain, often the area around the posterior superior iliac spine and sacroiliac joint is tender.
- The hip is too deep to palpate but feel around the greater trochanter for bursae.

Movement
- Assess movements of the spine. Diminished movement is likely if pathology is present. It may be impossible for the patient to comply because of pain.
- Hip movements will be reduced if an arthritic process is present. Usually internal rotation and abduction are the first to be lost.

Special tests
Straight leg raising will be diminished with a positive sciatic stretch test if the nerve root is irritated by a prolapsed disc or spinal stenosis.

A peripheral nervous system examination may show weakness and sensory loss in a single nerve root pattern.

Investigation of a patient with back, hip and leg pain
Blood tests
These are not always necessary but should be performed to exclude sinister causes in patients over 55 years of age or as guided by clinical suspicion.

Full blood count may reveal:
- Raised white cell count if infection is present such as in discitis.
- Anaemia in malignancy.

Biochemistry is required only to exclude abdominal causes and help confirm cases of malignancy.
- Erythrocyte sedimentation rate (ESR) and C-reactive protein (CRP) are elevated in infection and malignancy.
- Patients presenting with metastatic disease and an unknown primary need thorough investigation. Biopsy specimens should be taken at surgery.

Plain X-ray
This may show:
- Normal appearances in low back pain, prolapsed disc and even in malignancy or infection if early in the disease process (it is therefore not a good screening test and some departments have stopped routine spinal X-rays in young patients).
- Osteoarthritic changes in the hip and spine.
- A spondylolisthesis.
- Destruction of the vertebral body, classically the pedicle (winking owl sign) (Fig. 1.2), indicating malignancy.
- Fracture.
- Erosion of vertebral body around the disc due to infection.

Further special tests may be needed if there is doubt about the diagnosis or to plan surgery:
- Isotope bone scanning: hot spot in infection and malignancy.
- CT scanning: for looking at bony structures in detail, e.g. spondylolisthesis.
- Magnetic resonance imaging: useful for looking at soft tissue structures, including identification of disc prolapse and nerve root prior to surgery; and early detection of malignancy and infection.

Algorithms for the diagnosis and investigation of back, hip and leg pain and for the investigation of sinister back pain are provided in Figures 1.3 and 1.4.

Knee pain

Knee pain is a very common presenting complaint, accounting for over a third of all referrals to orthopaedic surgeons.

Differential diagnosis
- Osteoarthritis (see Ch. 8).
- Meniscal injuries (see Ch. 22).
- Ligament injury.
- Rheumatoid or other inflammatory arthritis (including crystal arthritis).
- Referred from hip or spine.
- Osteochondritis.
- Bursitis (see Ch. 24).
- Septic arthritis (see Ch. 16).
- Anterior knee pain/patellofemoral disorders.

History focusing on knee pain
The first thing to consider is the patient's age and occupation. A young athletic patient with a recent injury is unlikely to have rheumatoid arthritis (think

Fig. 1.2 Malignancy of the spine. The winking owl sign occurs when the pedicle is destroyed due to metastasis. The missing 'eye' represents bony destruction of the pedicle by tumour, so always look closely at the pedicles.

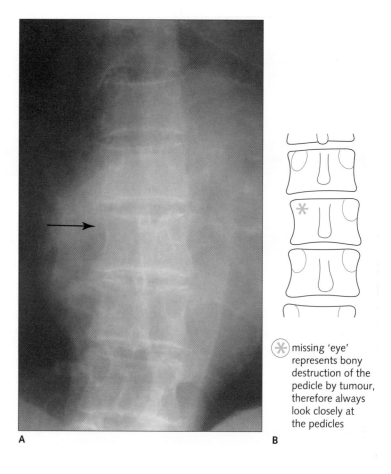

A   B

✳ missing 'eye' represents bony destruction of the pedicle by tumour, therefore always look closely at the pedicles

of meniscal/ligamentous injuries). Similarly an elderly patient with gradual onset of pain over many years will most likely have an arthritic process.

The characteristics of the pain will give clues to the underlying diagnosis.

Site of pain

Pain can be generalized or localized.

Generalized pain ('all over') suggests an arthritic process affecting the whole joint. Large effusions such as after an injury or in sepsis also give a tense painful joint.

Localized pain depends on the site. Commonly painful areas around the knee are shown in Figure 1.5.

- Anterior: patellofemoral pain is felt here. Pain is felt at the front of the knee in prepatellar and infrapatellar bursitis as well as the obvious diagnosis of anterior knee pain.
- Medial or lateral: localized pain to either joint line could be osteoarthritis (particularly so in varus

knees on the medial joint line) or from meniscal tears and collateral ligament sprains.

- Posterior pain is less common but could be related to a large Baker's cyst or bursitis.
- Pain down back of knee could be referred from the spine.
- Pain down the front of the thigh and into the knee suggests hip pathology.

The mode of onset is usually gradual, over a few weeks or months. If there is a sudden onset the most likely cause is an injury to the knee such as a meniscal tear or fracture. A history of spontaneous pain over days is most likely due to septic or crystal arthritis but could signal a flare-up of inflammatory conditions.

Pain and stiffness in the morning improving through the day suggest an inflammatory arthritis.

Pain originating from knee pathology rarely radiates but hip pain is commonly felt in the knee, particularly in children.

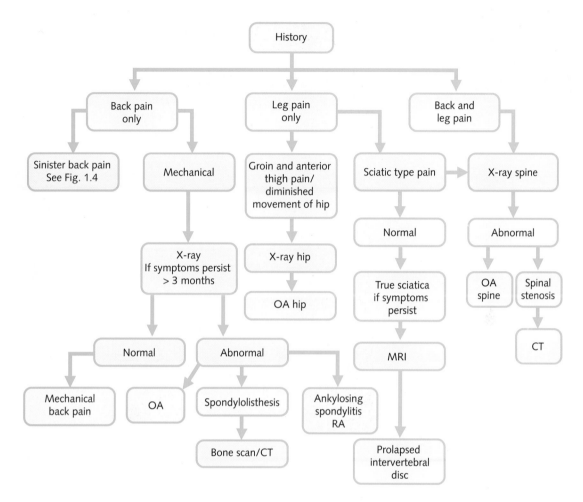

Fig. 1.3 Algorithm for the diagnosis and investigation of back, hip and leg pain. CT, computed tomography; MRI, magnetic resonance imaging; OA, osteoarthritis; RA, rheumatoid arthritis.

Nature of pain

Meniscal tear often gives a sharp stabbing pain.

Arthritic pain is usually a deep gnawing pain.

Constant pain that is not affected by activity is often a feature of anterior knee pain.

Aggravating factors/relieving factors

Arthritic pain is generally worse on activity and relieved by rest.

Classically patellofemoral pain is worse on walking up or down stairs.

Meniscal tears may give more trouble in deep flexion or when twisting.

In an acute crystal or septic arthritis the pain is intense and any movement exacerbates this considerably.

Pain from prepatellar bursitis is worse on kneeling.

Loss of function

Patients may have significant disability due to their knee pain. They may notice decreased movement or loss of full extension.

Athletic patients with a meniscal tear or cruciate ligament injury will tell you they don't trust the knee during certain sporting activities and may be unable to do them at all.

Deformity (see Ch. 5)

Patients with arthritis may notice that they are gradually becoming more 'bow legged' or 'knock

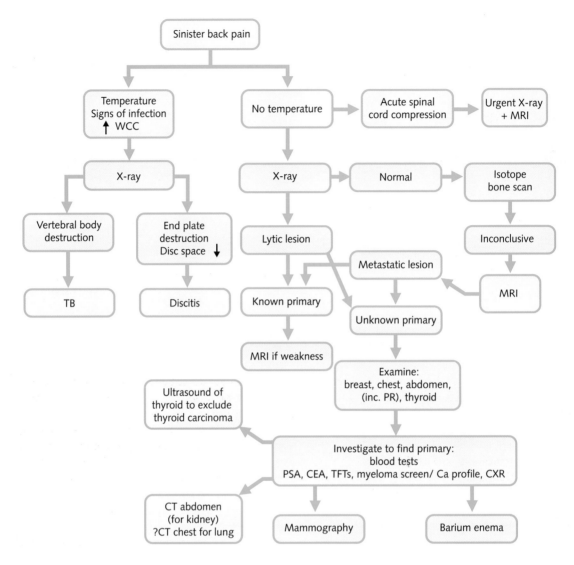

Fig. 1.4 Algorithm for the investigation of sinister back pain. Ca, calcium; CEA, carcinoembryonic antigen; CXR, chest X-ray; MRI, magnetic resonance imaging; PR, per rectum; PSA, prostate specific antigen; TFTs, thyroid function tests; WCC, white cell count.

kneed'. A windswept deformity (one valgus knee and one varus knee) is more common in rheumatoid arthritis (RA).

Associated symptoms

It is important to ask some closed questions when taking a history in a patient with knee pain.

Ask about any generalized symptoms of ill-health such as a fever.

Any history of injury is important, as often a sportsman/woman will ignore a knee injury for many years prior to seeking help. The anterior cruciate ligament (ACL) may have been torn, so take a detailed history about what happened.

- Ask if the patient heard a 'snap'.
- Ask how long the swelling took to appear (very sudden swelling suggests ACL rupture).
- Ask whether the patient could play on (unlikely if significant injury occurred).
- A history of locking suggests meniscal injury or loose body.
- Giving way may be due to a ligamentous problem such as ACL rupture.

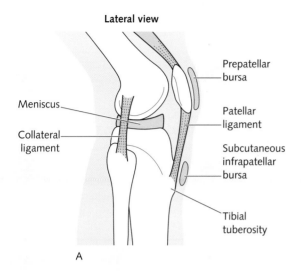

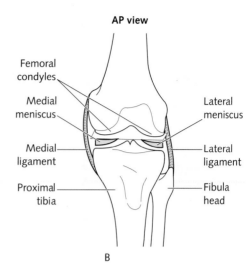

Fig. 1.5 Anatomical structures in the knee that cause pain.

Past medical history
Of particular interest will be any previous operations or fractures to the knee, such as meniscectomy or arthroscopy.

Drug history
Ask about medications such as analgesics and non-steroidal anti-inflammatory drugs (NSAIDs).

Examination
As with any orthopaedic examination, the principles are look, feel and move.

Remember to examine the other knee as a comparison. This will give you an idea of how lax they are normally (this varies considerably) and how much movement they have.

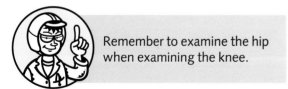

Remember to examine the hip when examining the knee.

General inspection could reveal signs of rheumatoid arthritis.

Watch the patient walk into the room, look for an antalgic or Trendelenburg gait.

Inspection
- Look at the patient on standing, as any deformity will be more obvious. A varus deformity is more common than a valgus one.
- Look for previous scars around the knee, wasting (particularly quadriceps), swelling and erythema.
- Swelling can be localized such as a prepatellar bursa (a boggy swelling in front of the knee) or more generalized such as an effusion.

Palpation
- Palpate for an effusion as described in Chapter 27.
- Palpate for tenderness around the knee; joint line tenderness is common in a patient with a meniscal tear. A meniscal cyst may also be found.
- Palpate behind the knee for a bursa or Baker's cyst.
- Patellofemoral crepitus can be felt (and sometimes heard) on flexing and extending the knee in osteoarthritis.

Movement
- A locked knee results in lack of full extension but often flexion is normal. This can be quite subtle so compare with the other side.
- Fixed flexion deformity (common in osteoarthritis) also causes loss of full extension but the history is more gradual.
- Arthritis results in variable amounts of decreased flexion.
- See if any deformity is correctable.

Special tests

- Collateral ligament tears are apparent on abnormal opening up of the joint on the affected side.
- Anterior cruciate ligament laxity is demonstrated by positive Lachmann's and anterior drawer tests.
- Posterior cruciate ligament laxity is seen as a sag of the tibia at 90° and can be misdiagnosed as an ACL tear when performing the anterior drawer test (the abnormal forward movement of the tibia is due to its sagging back in the first place).
- Maltracking of the patella can be seen when observing the knee bending from flexion to extension (so-called J sign).
- Patella apprehension will be positive in a patient with previous dislocation.

Investigations

Figure 1.6 provides an algorithm for the investigation of knee pain.

Blood tests

A full blood count (FBC) and measurements of ESR and CRP should be performed in suspected cases of infection and will show raised inflammatory markers and a high white cell count (WCC).

X-rays

X-ray images should be taken standing (joint space narrowing becomes more obvious) and include anteroposterior (AP), lateral and skyline views.

The X-ray may:
- Confirm rheumatoid arthritis or osteoarthritis.

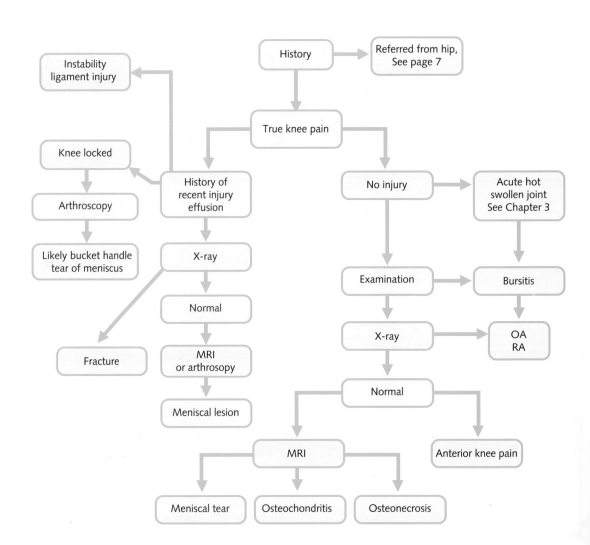

Fig. 1.6 Algorithm for the investigation of knee pain. MRI, magnetic resonance imaging; OA, osteoarthritis; RA, rheumatoid arthritis.

- Show a fracture.
- Be normal.

Remember to consider an X-ray of the hip based on your history and examination findings.

Further imaging

This is only warranted under certain conditions:

- Magnetic resonance imaging (MRI): useful to confirm meniscal or ligamentous pathology.
- Computed tomography (CT): gives detailed information on bony structures; also useful to visualize patellar tracking.
- Isotope bone scanning: occasionally used if unsure about diagnosis. It will show 'hot spots' due to increased activity in many conditions including osteoarthritis, but also rarer causes such as osteomyelitis and bone tumours. It is a sensitive test but not specific. A normal bone scan is reassuring if one suspects sinister pathology.

Aspiration

Aspiration of joint fluid is a very simple method of investigation and can give clues to the diagnosis.

Look at the fluid obtained:

- Straw/yellow fluid: likely to be a simple effusion or possibly a crystal arthropathy.
- Green or dirty fluid: likely to be pus, and septic arthritis is likely.
- Blood: a haemarthrosis occurs after injury or occasionally in bleeding disorders or patients on warfarin. Blood and fat globules (a lipohaemarthrosis; Fig. 1.7) are present in fracture or ACL rupture.

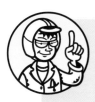
Always send fluid obtained to microbiology for microscopy, culture and sensitivities (M, C + S) and ask the laboratory to look for crystals.

Arthroscopy

Knee arthroscopy involves 'keyhole' surgery to look into the joint to see if there is any pathology. Such exploratory operations used to be very common but now most surgeons will have a clear idea about the diagnosis before operating in such a way.

Often, based on clinical findings, the surgeon is sure of the diagnosis and will operate without the need for further investigations such as MRI scanning. This is particularly true in a locked knee.

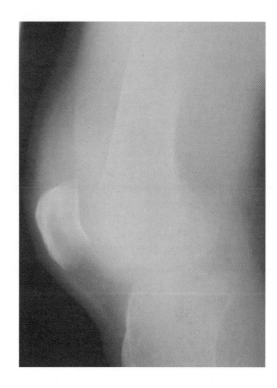

Fig. 1.7 A lipohaemarthrosis in the suprapatellar pouch. A fluid level is seen as the fat 'floats' on the blood.

Neck and/or upper limb pain

Differential diagnosis

Figures 1.8–1.11 give the differential diagnoses that should be considered when patients present with neck, shoulder, elbow, or wrist and hand pain.

Remember that pain in any bone or joint can be due to trauma, sepsis or malignancy.

Complex regional pain syndrome

This is also referred to as reflex sympathetic dystrophy, algodystrophy, or Sudeck's atrophy. It can affect any part of the musculoskeletal system. The distal forearm and hand are commonly involved, which is why the syndrome is included in this section. The key features are of pain, hypersensitivity and autonomic disturbances, which can affect the integrity of the skin.

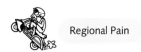

Differential diagnosis of neck pain
Mechanical neck pain
Cervical spondylosis
Cervical disc prolapse
Cervical discitis
Metastatic vertebral deposits
Referred pain from:
• Local structures (e.g. thyroiditis, cervical lymphadenopathy)
• Distant structures (e.g. ischaemic heart disease, subphrenic abscess)

Fig. 1.8 Differential diagnosis of neck pain.

Differential diagnosis of shoulder pain
Arthritis of the glenohumeral joint
Arthritis of the acromioclavicular (AC) joint
Rotator cuff tendinitis or degeneration
Rotator cuff tear
Bicipital tendinitis
Capsulitis
Polymyalgia rheumatica
Referred pain from:
• Neck pathology
• Cardiac ischaemia
• Pancoast's tumour
• Intra-abdominal pathology (e.g. subphrenic abscess)

Fig. 1.9 Differential diagnosis of shoulder pain.

Differential diagnosis of elbow pain
Lateral epicondylitis
Medial epicondylitis
Olecranon bursitis
Crystal arthropathy
Osteoarthritis
Referred pain from the neck or shoulder

Fig. 1.10 Differential diagnosis of elbow pain.

Differential diagnosis of pain in the hand and wrist
Osteoarthritis
Inflammatory arthritis
Crystal arthropathy
Tenosynovitis
Carpal tunnel syndrome
Ulnar nerve entrapment
Raynaud's phenomenon
Complex regional pain syndrome
Referred pain from the cervical spine, shoulder or elbow

Fig. 1.11 Differential diagnosis of pain in the hand and wrist.

History

The following points should be covered when taking a history from a patient with neck or upper limb pain:

Onset of pain

- Usually acute in cervical disc prolapse.
- Subacute in polymyalgia rheumatica or crystal arthropathy.
- Gradual in tendinitis, epicondylitis or degenerative joint disease.

History of recent trauma or strenuous activity

- A fall on an outstretched hand, particularly in an elderly person, may result in a Colles fracture or rotator cuff tear.
- Trauma can trigger complex regional pain syndrome.
- Unaccustomed repetitive upper limb use, such as painting a ceiling, may provoke tendinitis of the rotator cuff or wrist, or lateral epicondylitis.

The presence of any other precipitating factors

- Raynaud's phenomenon is provoked by cold weather.
- Acute gout may be precipitated by the introduction of drugs that affect the serum urate level.

Site of pain

- The site of pain may give a clue to its origin. Figure 1.12 shows how the site of shoulder pain varies with the cause.
- Capsulitis Carpal tunnel syndrome causes pain in the radial three and a half digits.

Movements that aggravate the pain

- Shoulder pain due to rotator cuff tendinitis will be exacerbated by abduction of the shoulder.
- Capsulitis causes pain on all shoulder movements.

Presence of associated symptoms

- Stiffness is found in inflammatory conditions such as inflammatory arthritis or polymyalgia rheumatica.
- Referral of neck pain to the upper limbs or the presence of paraesthesia may be due to cervical nerve root irritation.
- Weakness or clumsiness of the lower limbs or urinary symptoms may result from cervical cord compression.

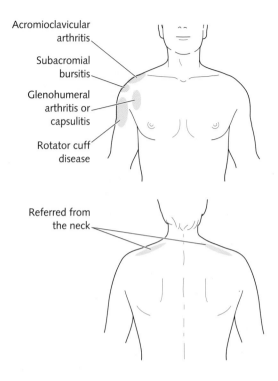

Acromioclavicular arthritis

Subacromial bursitis

Glenohumeral arthritis or capsulitis

Rotator cuff disease

Referred from the neck

Fig. 1.12 Many structures can give rise to shoulder pain. These diagrams show how the site of pain varies with the origin.

- Dizziness may occur as a result of vertebral artery compression in severe degenerative disease.
- Paraesthesia usually accompanies pain in median or ulnar nerve entrapment.
- A painful response to stimuli that do not usually cause pain (e.g. light touch) is called allodynia and occurs in complex regional pain syndrome.
- Fever, weight loss and general malaise raise the possibility of sepsis, malignancy or inflammatory conditions such as polymyalgia rheumatica.
- Some symptoms will give a clue to the presence of disease that may be causing referred pain (e.g. haemoptysis in a patient with a Pancoast's tumour).

A suggested algorithm for the examination and investigation of patients with neck and/or upper limb pain is shown in Figure 1.13.

Examination
Inspection
Inspection of the affected joint and surrounding area is important. This may reveal:

- Loss of the normal cervical lordosis due to cervical spondylosis or muscle spasm.
- Wasting of the shoulder muscles from chronic rotator cuff tendinitis.
- Shiny, erythematous swelling of the elbow or wrist due to acute gout or pseudogout.
- Synovial swelling of the small hand joints or tendon sheaths.
- Rheumatoid nodules.
- Plaques of psoriasis.
- Gouty tophi.
- Wasting of the thenar or hypothenar muscles resulting respectively from median or ulnar nerve compression.
- Ischaemic changes in the digits due to Raynaud's phenomenon.
- Changes in skin colour, with atrophy and reduced hair growth as features of complex regional pain syndrome.

Palpation
This helps in the assessment of swelling. Hard, bony swelling as seen in osteoarthritis should be distinguished from the softer, boggy, synovial swelling due to inflammatory arthritis. Tenderness of tendon insertions around the shoulder and elbow is suggestive of rotator cuff tendinitis or epicondylitis respectively. Inflamed tendon sheaths in the hand or wrist may feel thickened or nodular and palpation may produce crepitus.

Palpation of the neck should include the vertebral spinous processes, paravertebral muscles and occiput. Tenderness due to cervical spondylosis is often poorly localized. Extreme tenderness may be due to discitis or malignancy.

Assessment of joint movement
Assessment of joint movement is valuable in a hunt for the source of pain.

- In the shoulder, a reduction in passive and active movement suggests arthritis or capsulitis of the joint. A reduction in active movement, with normal passive movement, suggests a rotator cuff problem.
- Movement of the elbow in lateral epicondylitis will probably be normal, but resisted dorsiflexion of the wrist will exacerbate the pain.

Examination of other body systems
Neurological examination of the lower cranial nerves and all four limbs is essential in a patient with neck pain and any neurological symptoms. Cervical

13

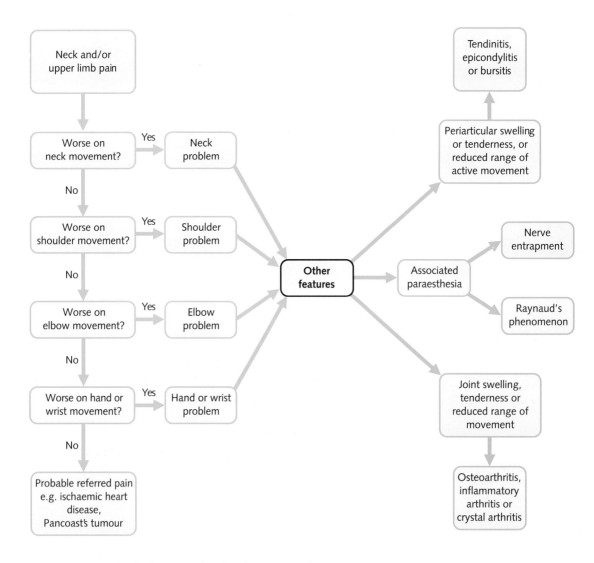

Fig. 1.13 Algorithm for the diagnosis of neck and/or upper limb pain.

radiculopathy and cord compression should be excluded. Motor and sensory function of the median and ulnar nerves should be assessed in cases of hand and wrist pain (Fig. 1.14). Tinel's and Phalen's tests may be abnormal in carpal tunnel syndrome.

Examination of the cardiovascular, respiratory and abdominal systems may reveal a source of referred pain.

Investigations

The choice of investigations depends on the clinical examination findings. In some cases, the diagnosis is obvious from examination and further investigation is not required. For example, a 75-year-old man who

complains of pain in his digits and has squaring of his first carpometacarpal joint and Heberden's nodes has osteoarthritis. Plain X-rays will confirm the diagnosis, but will not alter his management in any way.

Blood tests
- Erythrocyte sedimentation rate (ESR) and C-reactive protein (CRP) will be raised in inflammatory, infectious or malignant conditions.
- The finding of a positive rheumatoid factor in a patient with synovitis is suggestive of rheumatoid arthritis.
- Serum uric acid is likely to be raised in cases of gout.

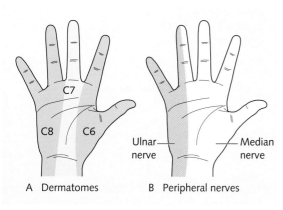

Fig. 1.14 Nerve entrapment in the upper limb can cause pain, paraesthesia or sensory loss in the hand. The digit(s) affected give a clue as to which nerve is involved.

Synovial fluid examination
- Polarized light microscopy may detect urate or calcium pyrophosphate crystals.
- Microscopy and culture should be performed if there is any suspicion of infection.

Radiological investigations
X-rays
Plain X-rays may show signs of:
- Degenerative or inflammatory arthritis.
- Calcification due to tendinitis.
- Periosteal reaction due to enthesitis.
- Bony metastasis.

 X-rays are of little value in cervical spondylosis. There is poor correlation between the severity of radiographic signs and symptoms. Many people develop radiographic signs of spondylosis with increasing age, yet never suffer from neck pain.

Ultrasound scans
Ultrasound scanning can demonstrate thickening and oedema of tendon sheaths in tenosynovitis.

MRI and CT scans
These are useful in the following circumstances:
- Imaging the cervical cord and nerve roots.
- Detecting rotator cuff inflammation or degeneration.

Isotope bone scans
Isotope bone scans show increased tracer uptake in areas of accelerated bone turnover, such as infection, malignancy or fracture. The finding of a 'hot spot' should be followed by MRI or CT scanning.

Nerve conduction studies
These can help to exclude cervical radiculopathy in patients with neck pain and upper limb paraesthesia. Those with abnormal nerve conduction should proceed to an MRI or CT scan. Reduced nerve conduction velocities are seen in median and ulnar nerve entrapment.

Ankle and foot pain

Differential diagnosis
The differential diagnosis of pain in the ankle and/or foot is shown in Figure 1.15.

 Remember that pain in any bone or joint can be due to trauma, sepsis or malignancy.

History
The following points should be covered when taking a history from patients with ankle or foot pain:

Site and chronological pattern of pain
(see Fig. 1.15)
- Recurrent self-limiting pain suggests inflammation (e.g. gout).
- Chronic pain with soft-tissue swelling suggests inflammation or infection.
- Pain on standing or walking suggests arthritis or a biomechanical problem.
- Pain on effort (running, prolonged walking) suggests a biomechanical problem.

Presence of associated symptoms
- Stiffness is common in inflammatory conditions.
- Back or knee pain suggest that the pain may be referred.

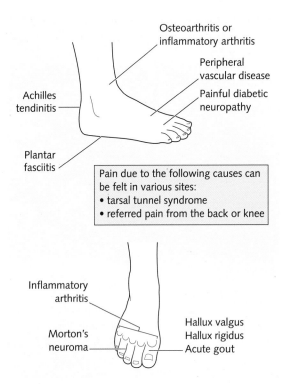

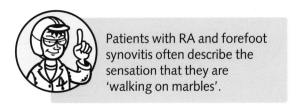

Fig. 1.15 Differential diagnosis of ankle and/or foot pain.

- Coldness and pallor of the foot may be due to peripheral vascular disease.
- Paraesthesia or 'burning' pain can occur with Morton's neuroma, painful diabetic neuropathy or tarsal tunnel syndrome.

Detailed past medical history
- Plantar fasciitis is associated with spondyloarthropathies, so ask about a history of psoriasis or inflammatory bowel disease.
- Primary osteoarthritis (OA) is rare in the ankle or subtalar joints, so OA at these sites is usually secondary to previous ankle instability or fracture.
- Diabetes mellitus may be complicated by a painful neuropathy.
- Smoking, hypertension and diabetes mellitus are risk factors for peripheral vascular disease.

Presence of any precipitating factors
- Repetitive trauma due to running, jumping or other athletic activities can predispose to Achilles tendinitis, pre-Achilles bursitis or 'Policeman's heel'.
- A recent illness or initiation of diuretic therapy may trigger an acute attack of gout.

Examination

The ankle and foot should be inspected during weight bearing as well as in the neutral position. Some clinical signs are more obvious when the patient is standing.

Inspection
Inspection of the foot and ankle may reveal the following signs:
- Calluses under metatarsal joints (chronic biomechanical foot problems or arthritis).
- Valgus deformity at the first metatarsophalangeal (MTP) joint (hallux valgus).
- Erythematous swelling of the joint (acute gout or inflammatory arthritis).
- Swelling in the region of the Achilles tendon (Achilles tendinitis).
- Ischaemic changes due to peripheral vascular disease.
- Plaques of psoriasis.

Palpation
Palpation of the foot and ankle should assess the following:
- Swelling, is it bony or soft?
- Joint tenderness.
- Tenderness of the plantar fascia and Achilles tendon.
- Tenderness between the metatarsal heads and/or the nodular swelling of a Morton's neuroma.
- Tenderness over the posterior tibial nerve posterior to the medial malleolus (common in tarsal tunnel syndrome).
- Strength of the peripheral pulses.

Movement
Movement of the foot and ankle should be compared to that on the opposite side. Passive dorsiflexion of

the ankle will exacerbate the pain of Achilles tendonitis. Restriction of movement and crepitus of the first MTP joint is seen with hallux rigidus.

Examination of other joints
This must include the knee, hip and lumbar spine.

Neurological examination
Neurological examination of the lower limbs is essential if there is any suspicion that the pain might be referred from the lumbar spine. Sensation should be tested. Diabetic neuropathy will cause sensory loss in a stocking distribution, whereas in Morton's neuroma it is localized to the borders of adjacent toes. The site of anaesthesia in tarsal tunnel syndrome depends on which branch of the posterior tibial nerve is compressed.

Investigations
Blood tests
- The ESR and CRP will be elevated in most cases of inflammatory arthritis and crystal arthropathy.
- Serum uric acid levels are usually raised during acute attacks of gout.

- The finding of a positive rheumatoid factor in a patient with synovitis is suggestive of rheumatoid arthritis.

Radiological investigations
- Plain X-rays may show signs of an inflammatory or degenerative arthritis.
- Ultrasonography can identify abnormalities of the Achilles tendon and Morton's neuromas.
- Magnetic resonance imaging (MRI) can also be used to assess tendons and neuromas. MRI of the lumbosacral spine is the investigation of choice in patients with ankle or foot pain that is thought to be due to nerve root compression.

Synovial fluid examination
Synovial fluid examination under polarized light microscopy should be performed if there are any pointers to a crystal arthropathy, such as acute erythema, pain and swelling in the first metatarsophalangeal joint or ankle.

Nerve conduction studies
These are useful in confirming the diagnosis of tarsal tunnel syndrome or peripheral neuropathy.

Fig. 2.2 Algorithm for the investigation of widespread musculoskeletal pain. ANA, antinuclear antibody; CRP, C-reactive protein; ESR, erythrocyte sedimentation rate; PMR, polymyalgia rheumatica; SLE, systemic lupus erythematosus.

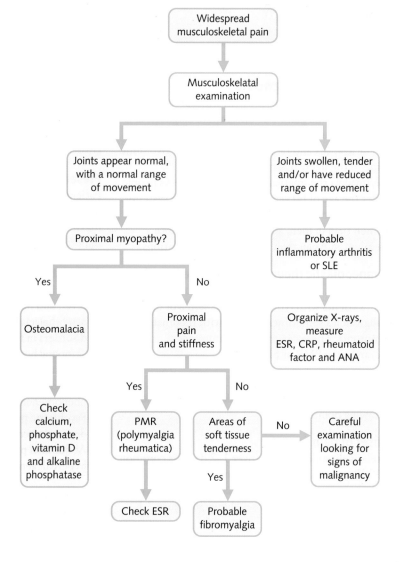

repeated if symptoms persist. For example, the radiological signs of inflammatory arthritis may take months to appear.

Blood tests

- The ESR is likely to be raised in cases of PMR, inflammatory arthritis, SLE or malignancy.
- Serum calcium levels may be low in osteomalacia.
- Parathyroid hormone levels should be checked in the presence of hypercalcaemia to exclude hyperparathyroidism.
- Serum alkaline phosphatase may be elevated in osteomalacia. It can also rise in response to inflammation.
- An immunology screen, including measurement of antinuclear and anti-double-stranded DNA antibodies and immunoglobulin levels, will be abnormal in active SLE.
- Rheumatoid factor is found in the serum of up to 90% of patients with rheumatoid arthritis.

Radiological investigations

X-rays of the small joints may show the erosive changes of inflammatory arthritis. Radiographs of the long bones and pelvis should be taken if the patient has risk factors for osteomalacia, such as reduced sunlight exposure or intestinal malabsorption. Looser's zones may be seen.

Other radiological tests (e.g. chest X-ray, abdominal ultrasound scan) may be necessary if there is any suspicion of malignancy.

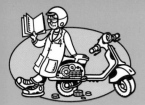

3. An Acute Hot Swollen Joint

Differential diagnosis

- Septic arthritis
- Crystal synovitis
  —Gout
  —Pseudogout
- Rheumatoid or other inflammatory arthritis (including Reiter's syndrome)
- Reactive arthritis
- Haemarthrosis.

The phrase 'acute hot swollen joint' implies that the patient has presented as an emergency with rapid onset of symptoms and a large painful effusion.

History focusing on the acute hot swollen joint

Pain

Patients with acute gout or septic arthritis classically have very severe pain. However, it is difficult to differentiate these conditions from other causes of hot swollen joints as the majority of patients will present with intense pain that is worse on movement.

Patient age and sex

All of the above conditions could present in the adult patient, whereas only septic arthritis, reactive arthritis and possibly inflammatory arthritis are likely causes in children.

Gout is more common in men, and rheumatoid arthritis is more common in women.

Pseudogout is usually found in the elderly, with gout more common in young and middle-aged adults.

Which joint?

Certain joints are more commonly affected by specific disorders (Fig. 3.1):

- Gout commonly affects the first metatarsophalangeal (MTP) joint of the foot.
- Pseudogout is common in the knee and wrist.
- Multiple joint involvement points to an inflammatory disorder such as rheumatoid arthritis (RA) or juvenile idiopathic arthritis (JIA).

Is the patient ill?

Fever, night sweats, rigors and general flu-like symptoms suggest likely infection *but* it is possible to have the same symptoms in an acute 'flare-up' of an inflammatory arthropathy.

Previous history

This is likely in gout as 90% of patients with an acute attack will have recurrent episodes.

It is unlikely in septic arthritis unless the patient has a predisposing factor such as sickle cell disease (see Ch. 16).

Be careful! Patients with known inflammatory or crystal arthritis can present with an infected joint.

Associated symptoms

Patients with an inflammatory disorder may have systemic features of the disease process such as sacroiliac joint pain in ankylosing spondylitis or painful metacarpophalangeal (MCP) joints in RA.

Eye symptoms can occur in:

- Reiter's syndrome (conjunctivitis)
- Rheumatoid arthritis (keratoconjunctivitis)
- Juvenile idiopathic arthritis (uveitis).

Patients with a history of recent sexually transmitted disease or diarrhoea are likely to have Reiter's syndrome.

Also consider gonococcal arthritis in patients with a history of sexually transmitted diseases (STDs).

A recent viral illness can result in a reactive arthritis.

Past medical history

Gout is linked with increased cell turnover and therefore any illness can predispose to it due to increase in breakdown products.

Patients with malignancy having chemotherapy are particularly prone to gout due to vast numbers of cells being 'killed' (see Ch. 13).

As mentioned in Chapter 16, certain conditions also predispose to joint infection, e.g. intravenous drug use (IVDU).

Patients with a bleeding disorder (such as haemophilia) or on warfarin are at risk of developing an acute haemarthrosis (bleeding into a joint). These patients can present in such a way with an acutely swollen tender joint.

Fig. 3.1 Likely diagnosis for each joint in a patient presenting with an acute hot swollen joint.

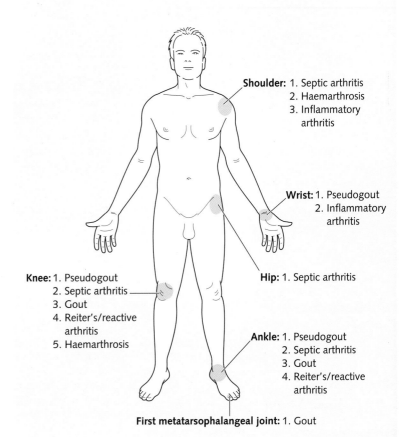

Shoulder: 1. Septic arthritis
2. Haemarthrosis
3. Inflammatory arthritis

Wrist: 1. Pseudogout
2. Inflammatory arthritis

Hip: 1. Septic arthritis

Knee: 1. Pseudogout
2. Septic arthritis
3. Gout
4. Reiter's/reactive arthritis
5. Haemarthrosis

Ankle: 1. Pseudogout
2. Septic arthritis
3. Gout
4. Reiter's/reactive arthritis

First metatarsophalangeal joint: 1. Gout

Drug history

Diuretics and aspirin can increase uric acid levels, predisposing to gout.

Patients on steroids or other immunosuppressants are at increased risk of infection.

Social history

The effects of 'bad living' (rich diet and alcohol) as a cause of gout have been overstated in the past but may play a role.

Examination of a patient with an acute hot swollen joint
General

- Most patients presenting in such a way will look unwell, be uncomfortable and may be agitated.
- A pyrexia suggests infection but mildly elevated temperatures can be present in gout and inflammatory arthritis.
- The patient should be examined for general signs of inflammatory arthritis.

- Patients with gout may have gouty tophi; these are commonly found on extensor surfaces of the elbow and fingers.

The joint

- The knee is the most commonly affected joint overall.
- Any affected joint will have a tense effusion and be exquisitely tender to any passive movement.
- A full examination of the joint is unnecessary and impossible!
- A thorough examination of other joints should be performed to make sure the patient has a monoarthritis (i.e. no other joints are involved!).

Investigation of a patient with an acute swollen joint

An algorithm for the investigation of a patient with an acute swollen joint is shown in Figure 3.2.

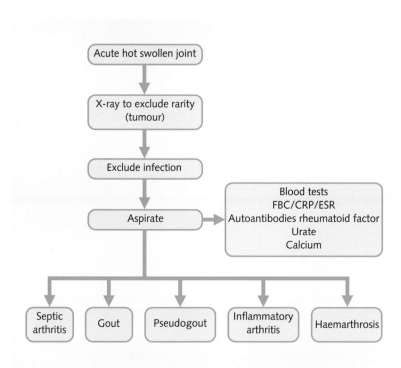

Fig. 3.2 Algorithm for the investigation of an acute hot swollen joint. CRP, C-reactive protein; ESR, erythrocyte sedimentation rate; FBC, full blood count.

Blood tests

The aim of initial investigation is to confirm or exclude septic arthritis as this condition needs prompt treatment to avoid irreparable damage to the joint.

- A raised white cell count (WCC) suggests infection.
- Inflammatory markers C-reactive protein (CRP) and erythrocyte sedimentation rate (ESR) can be raised in all the conditions listed above, particularly septic arthritis and inflammatory arthritis.

Normal inflammatory markers cannot completely exclude infection.

- Serum urate may be elevated, normal or low in patients with acute gout.
- Serum calcium should be checked as pseudogout can be caused by hyperparathyroidism.
- If haemarthrosis is suspected a clotting screen should be performed and patients on warfarin should have their international normalized ratio (INR) checked.

X-rays

Plain X-rays of the affected joint may show:

- Normal appearances.
- Chondrocalcinosis (found in pseudogout due to calcium deposition in menisci).

- Rheumatoid arthritis.
- Bony erosions associated with gout.

Of all the investigations the most important is aspiration of the joint.

Aspiration/synovial fluid analysis

- A superficial joint such as the knee is simple to aspirate, particularly when there is a tense effusion.
- Deeply situated joints such as the hip require ultrasound or X-ray guidance.
- In every case fluid aspirated must be sent to microbiology for urgent microscopy, culture and sensitivity (usually written as M, C and S). In addition to this the technician should look for crystals.
- The general appearance of the aspirate should be described (see Chs 1 and 30).

Ultrasound

Ultrasound scanning is useful to detect an effusion, particularly in the hip.

4. A Child With a Limp

Differential diagnosis
- Irritable hip.
- Developmental dysplasia of the hip (DDH).
- Perthes disease.
- Slipped upper femoral epiphysis (SUFE).
- Septic arthritis.
- Osteomyelitis.
- Occult trauma.
- Neuromuscular causes.
- Juvenile idiopathic arthritis.
- Malignancy (very rare).

History focusing on the child with a limp
There is a big difference between an infant aged 15 months and an adolescent aged 15 years. Infants will not give an accurate history and if very unwell may be distressed and uncooperative. The majority of children do, however, give a good history.

Age
The most important factor in assessing a child with a limp is the age of the child. Figure 4.1 shows the likely differential diagnosis depending on the age of the child.

Sex
The sex of the child can also give clues to the diagnosis; for example, Perthes disease is much more common in boys than in girls.

Is the child ill?
To answer this question the general state of the child must be noted. Systemically unwell children will show little interest in play or food and simply will not be themselves. Fever, rigors and night sweats should be noted as well as duration of symptoms. An unwell child suggests infection or juvenile idiopathic arthritis (JIA).

Pain
Most children limp because of pain.

Any child complaining of knee pain must be suspected of having hip pathology.

The history in Perthes disease is often of a vague gradual onset of pain and limp.

More sudden onset of pain is more likely due to trauma or infection.

The classic history for a slipped upper femoral epiphysis is often a background of hip pain for weeks followed by sudden increase in pain.

Transient synovitis of the hip gives pain in the groin and mimics septic arthritis.

Occasionally sinister causes of pain (such as bone tumours) present with gradually increasing pain (including night pain) not relieved by simple analgesia.

Painless limp
- Late-presenting DDH presents with limp and leg length discrepancy.

Diagnosis by age in a child with a limp	
All ages	Infection (septic arthritis or osteomyelitis) Juvenile idiopathic arthritis
Infant (1–3 years)	late-presenting developmental dysplasia of the hip (DDH) Irritable hip Neuromuscular Occult trauma (including non-accidental injury)
Childhood (3–11 years)	Perthes disease Irritable hip Neuromuscular Slipped upper femoral epiphysis (SUFE) Non-accidental injury (NAI)
Adolescence (12–16 years)	SUFE Infection

Fig. 4.1 Diagnosis by age in a child with a limp.

- Neuromuscular disorders such as cerebral palsy result in poor gait due to muscle imbalance rather than pain.
- Cerebral palsy can present as developmental delay but milder forms can present later in childhood as the weakness becomes more apparent.
- Muscular dystrophy can also present with gradual onset of weakness and limp.

Associated symptoms

History of injury may be elicited in occult trauma but in non-accidental injury (NAI) this will not be forthcoming.

Multiple joint aches and pains suggest juvenile arthritis.

A recent history of upper respiratory tract infection (URTI) or otitis media is often found in patients with transient synovitis.

In JIA the eyes can be involved as part of the systemic effects of the disease. If left untreated blindness can result.

Past medical history

Any previous history of Perthes disease or slipped upper femoral epiphysis (SUFE) is very important as these patients are at increased risk of developing disease in the opposite hip.

Family history

A family history of Perthes disease and DDH also leads to an increased risk.

Examining a child with a limp
General

Systemic features of ill-health such as pyrexia, drowsiness and irritability should be noted and will point towards infection as the cause.

Multiple joint problems may be obvious initially, suggesting juvenile idiopathic arthritis.

Neuromuscular disorders may be obvious or detected on neurological examination.

Inspection
Gait

- An antalgic gait is present in painful conditions such as Perthes or irritable hip.
- A Trendelenburg gait (see Ch. 27) is present in a toddler with late DDH.
- Neuromuscular disorders give a variety of patterns of gait abnormality.
- A worrying sign is a child too ill or in too much pain to weight bear.

Standing

- An abnormal single large posterior skin crease is present in DDH.
- In slipped upper femoral epiphysis or infection, the hip is often held in an abnormal position of external rotation and flexion (Fig. 4.2).

Further inspection could reveal scars, swelling or erythema.

Fixed flexion

If the Thomas test is positive (a fixed flexion deformity) suspect significant pathology such as advanced Perthes, DDH or SUFE.

Limb length discrepancy

- A short leg is typical of DDH.
- Apparent shortening (see Ch. 27) will be present if there is any fixed deformity.

Palpation

Palpate any tender areas for effusion, warmth and localized pain.

Tenderness over the tibial tubercle is likely to be due to Osgood–Schlatter disease.

Palpation around the knee will reveal joint line tenderness in conditions such as osteochondritis or, in older children, meniscal tears.

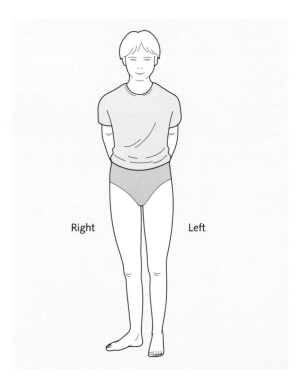

Fig. 4.2 External rotation deformity: child with externally rotated leg in slipped upper femoral epiphysis.

Movement

- Loss of hip movements indicates pathology.
- DDH results in loss of abduction compared with the other side.
- Perthes disease results in loss of abduction and flexion. Complete loss of abduction is a worrying sign in Perthes as this may indicate subluxation of the joint.
- In septic arthritis any movement gives extreme pain.

Investigating a child with a limp

Figure 4.3 provides an algorithm for the investigation of a child with a limp.

Blood tests

Markedly raised white cell count (WCC), erythrocyte sedimentation rate (ESR) and C-reactive protein (CRP) are present in infection but these inflammatory markers can also be mildly increased in synovitis or JIA.

Very rare causes of abnormal blood tests include leukaemia.

X-rays

A plain X-ray is often unnecessary in the younger child, particularly in cases of transient synovitis.

A hip radiograph may show:
- A dislocated hip.
- Perthes disease.
- A slipped upper femoral epiphysis.
- Evidence of infection (remember X-rays are initially normal).
- A fracture.

If slipped upper femoral epiphysis is suspected, request a frog lateral X-ray.

If you are sure the problem is from the knee then anteroposterior (AP) and lateral knee X-rays should be performed and may show:
- Osgood–Schlatter disease.
- Osteochondritis dissecans.
- A fracture.

Ultrasound

Ultrasound is a very useful investigation for suspected joint problems, particularly of the hip, which is deeply situated.

The scan will show an effusion in:
- Septic arthritis.
- Transient synovitis.
- Perthes disease (early).

Isotope bone scanning

If hot, this is likely to be significant and possible causes are:
- Osteomyelitis—the scan will also show any seeding of infection.
- Malignancy.

Magnetic resonance imaging (MRI)

MRI is not a first-line investigation in children but is useful in:
- Diagnosis of knee disorders (see Ch. 22).
- Bone and soft tissue tumours.
- Osteomyelitis.

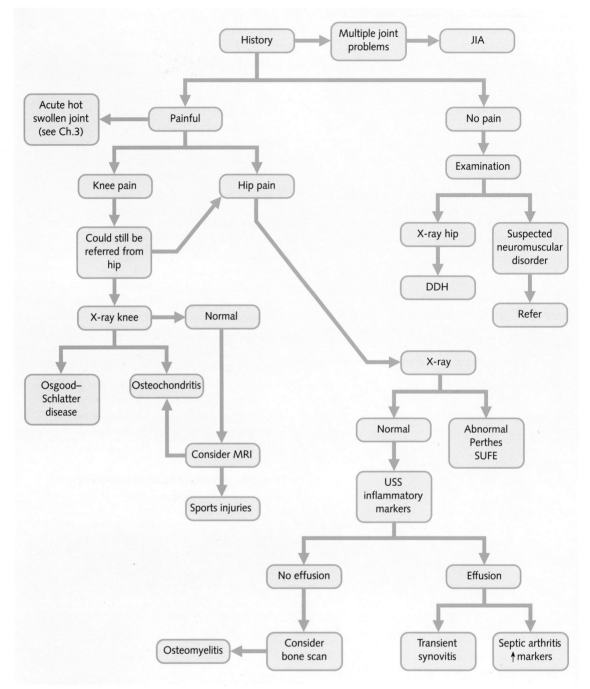

Fig. 4.3 Algorithm for the investigation of a child with a limp. DDH, developmental dysplasia of the hip; JIA, juvenile idiopathic arthritis; SUFE, slipped upper femoral epiphysis; USS, ultrasound scan.

5. Deformity

Definition
A deformity is due to an abnormal alignment or appearance of bone, joint or soft tissues.

A deformity can be correctable (able to return to original position) or fixed.
- Valgus deformity—bent away from the midline.
- Varus deformity—bent towards the midline.

Valgus and varus deformities of the knee are illustrated in Figure 5.1.

Causes of deformity
There are many causes of deformity and rather than list all of them the different causes have been listed as three groups, as follows:
1. Soft tissue:
   —Scarring
   —Swelling
   —Wasting
   —Overgrowth, e.g. Dupuytren's contracture.
2. Bone:
   a. Congenital
   b. Acquired:
      —Previous fracture
      —Infection
      —Tumours
      —Metabolic bone disease, e.g. sabre tibia in Paget's disease
      —Growth plate injury.
3. Joint:
   —Contracture (e.g. Volkmann's ischaemic contracture)
   —Muscle imbalance (e.g. polio)
   —Chronic arthritis (varus knee in osteoarthritis).

History focusing on deformity
Patients present with deformities for different reasons:
- Pain (usually associated with arthritic conditions).
- Disability (e.g. shortening of limb).
- Appearance (e.g. scoliosis).

Deformities in children are usually noted by the parents and often these patients have normal variations of growth and simply need reassurance (see Ch. 14).

It is important to recognize whether the deformity is due to a generalized disease process or only affects one limb.

An important initial question would be to ask if any other joints or limbs are involved.

Congenital deformities
Congenital deformities usually present at birth and are noted at delivery, although some will now be picked up on antenatal scanning.

An obstetric, birth and family history (the deformity could be present in siblings or either parent) should be noted.

Patients (or parents, if a child) will usually tell you they have 'had it since birth'.

If this is the case ask what has changed to make the patient seek help now.

The deformity may have progressed or become painful.

Cerebral palsy produces variable clinical deformities as the child grows.

Late presentation of developmental dysplasia of the hip (DDH; see Ch. 14) can occur, in which case the child will present with a limp when walking.

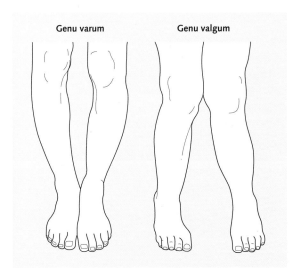

Genu varum   **Genu valgum**

Fig. 5.1 Genu varum and genu valgum.

Acquired deformities
Post-fracture, injury or sepsis

As a general rule deformities resulting from injuries are unilateral (i.e. you usually only injure one limb) and deformities from arthritis are bilateral (e.g. hand disease in rheumatoid arthritis is almost always bilateral).

This is usually progressive unilateral deformity following a specific injury.

Patients can often 'manage' very well with severe deformity until many years after an injury and then present with pain as secondary osteoarthritis becomes symptomatic.

Painful deformities
A painful deformity suggests an arthritic process but the patient is much more likely to present with pain before deformity becomes apparent. Typical deformities are varus knees and Heberden's nodes in osteoarthritis.

Paget's disease can also present with painful deformity.

Painless deformity
Painless deformity is common with neurological causes (such as ulna claw hand) or in Dupuytren's disease.

Such conditions affecting the hand can cause significant disability due to loss of function. For example the patient may be unable to hold tools for work.

Following a cerebrovascular accident (CVA) a patient has deformity due to muscle spasticity.

Loss of function
There is a wide variation in the effects of the deformity on function. Simple things such as being unable to wear a pair of shoes because of toe deformities can cause significant disability. Patients with severe Dupuytren's disease have difficulty combing their hair (sometimes poking themselves in the eye!).

Appearance
Often patients simply complain about the appearance of the deformity.

Scoliosis causes a prominent rib hump which is unsightly, and as most patients are of adolescent age significant distress results. If very severe, spinal deformity can result in chest complications due to decreased expansion.

One of the most common deformities seen is hallux valgus (bunions) and patients may 'only' complain that they have difficulty finding shoes to fit (not a good reason to operate)!

Associated symptoms
Generalized joint swelling and pain with deformity suggest inflammatory arthropathy.

Progression of deformity
The timing of events is important in assessing a patient with a deformity. Patients may have had the deformity for some years prior to presenting usually because there has been sudden progression or interference with day-to-day activities.

Examination of a patient with a deformity
There are features common to all deformities but the majority involve assessment of a limb or digit as described in Chapter 27.

Is the deformity correctable?
A deformity can be fixed or mobile.
- A mobile deformity will return to its original position when stressed. Only joint deformities can be mobile; an example is early varus deformity in osteoarthritis of the knee.
- A fixed deformity will not return to the original position. Most deformities are fixed. An example of a fixed deformity is a malunited tibial fracture.

Some conditions can be either fixed or mobile, such as hammer toe which can also be partially correctable.

Is there an associated condition?
Examine the whole patient to look for any generalized conditions associated with deformities such as an inflammatory arthritis.
- A patient with rheumatoid arthritis (RA) may have several typical deformities (usually in the hand).
- Patients with psoriatic arthropathy often present with very severe hand deformities (arthritis mutilans).
- A patient with cerebral palsy needs regular assessment, as deformity due to muscle imbalance can lead to fixed deformity and secondary bone changes. Common deformities in cerebral palsy include equinus of the foot and fixed flexion of the hip.

Common joint deformities

We will now look at each joint, looking for common deformities.

Hand

Examination of the hand may show:

- Thickened palmar fascia with fixed flexion deformity of the proximal interphalangeal (PIP) and metacarpophalangeal (MCP) joints (most commonly of the little and ring fingers), indicating Dupuytren's disease (Fig. 5.2).
- Heberden's nodes in osteoarthritis.
- Ulnar drift of the MCP joint, boutonnière deformity and swan-neck deformity, indicating rheumatoid arthritis
- Ulnar claw hand.

Elbow

The most important deformities at the elbow are cubitus valgus and cubitus varus (Fig. 5.3) and they are usually secondary to childhood fractures (supracondylar fracture of the elbow).

Shoulder

- A dislocated shoulder results in an abnormal contour (see Ch. 22).
- A winged scapula results from a long thoracic nerve palsy and the scapula is lifted off the chest wall on pushing forward.

Spine

- A torticollis (muscle spasm of the sternocleidomastoid muscle) causes the head to turn to the affected side.

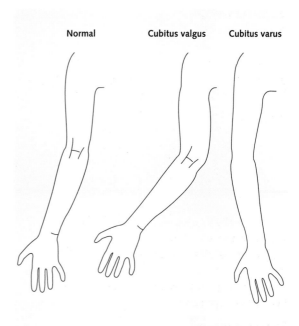

Fig. 5.3 Normal angle of the elbow, cubitus valgus and cubitus varus.

- A kyphosis is a flexion deformity of the spine (Fig. 5.4).
- A scoliosis is a lateral and rotational curvature of the spine.

Hip

- Hip conditions may present with leg length discrepancy.

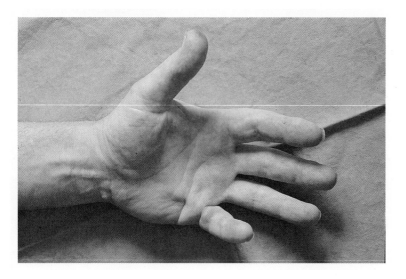

Fig. 5.2 Dupuytren's contracture of the palmar fascia (from Klippel J H, Dieppe P A (eds) 1998 Rheumatology, 2nd edn. Mosby, London).

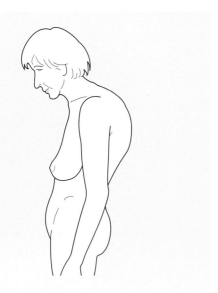

Fig. 5.4 A thoracic kyphosis.

- Fixed flexion of the hip gives patients an abnormal posture with the knee flexed and they often stoop to the affected side.

Knee
The knee is one of the most common sites for obvious clinical deformity.
- Varus or valgus knees can be constitutional (inherited) or secondary to degenerative change.
- Fixed flexion deformity of the knee results in loss of full extension and commonly occurs in osteoarthritis.

Foot and ankle
Deformities of the foot and ankle are also common (Figs 5.5 and 5.6). Common deformities of the forefoot are shown in Figure 27.23 (p. 188).

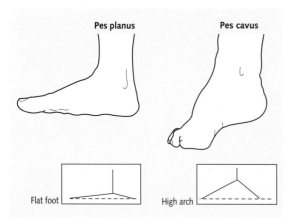

Fig. 5.5 Features of pes planus and pes cavus.

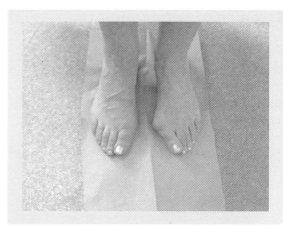

Fig. 5.6 Hallux valgus (bunions): right post- and left pre-operation. Note that the great toe is also pronated.

Investigation of a deformity
The majority of simple deformities need little or no investigation.
- Blood tests. It is unlikely, but a patient with inflammatory arthropathy could present in such a way. In this case check erythrocyte sedimentation rate (ESR), C-reactive protein (CRP), rheumatoid factor (RhF), autoantibodies.
- Abnormal biochemistry is present in Paget's disease (see Ch. 12).
- X-rays. The joint or limb involved will usually require X-ray examination. Special X-rays of the whole lower limb are needed for complex deformities.
- Nerve conduction studies are useful in assessing deformity secondary to peripheral nerve injury, e.g. ulna claw hand.
- Computed tomography (CT) scans are sometimes used to reconstruct complex deformities (3-D CT reconstruction).

6. A Limb Swelling

Differential diagnosis

It is helpful to consider differential diagnoses in relation to the anatomical location.

- Skin or subcutaneous:
  —Rheumatoid nodule
  —Lipoma
  —Bursitis
  —Neurofibroma
  —Cyst
- Joint:
  —Joint effusion
  —Ganglion
  —Baker's cyst
- Bone:
  —Bone tumour
- Muscle/deep soft tissues:
  —Sarcoma

Patients commonly present with lumps, bumps and swellings. The majority of these are benign, but it is important not to overlook very rare tumours presenting in this way.

History focusing on a swelling

The following points are important:

Duration of symptoms
How long has the patient had the lump or swelling, and when did the patient first notice it?

Increase in size
Has it increased in size recently or grown rapidly? Tumours may present in this way.

Solitary or multiple
Does the patient have more than one lump or swelling and if so where? Neurofibromata or rheumatoid nodules are often multiple.

Variability
Does the swelling come and go and if so over how long? Classically a ganglion will disappear and then recur.

Is it painful?
A tense effusion will be painful, as may bursitis. Deep pain related to a bony or soft tissue mass may be sinister. The majority of such lesions are not painful.

Loss of function
Does the swelling or lump inhibit the patient in any way. Swellings around the hand can be a nuisance to patients and those on the foot can rub when shoes are worn.

Associated symptoms
Usually there will be none.

The general health of the patient should be ascertained with weight loss, fatigue and poor health being sinister symptoms.

Occasionally large swelling or masses can compress vessels or nerves, e.g. osteochondroma.

Patients presenting with joint swelling may have other symptoms related to the underlying disease process, such as pain in the joint if arthritic.

A patient may have painless joint swelling as a presenting feature of a more generalized inflammatory condition. It is important therefore to ask about other joints such as those in the hand.

A patient with a Baker's cyst may have pain in the knee.

Occupational history
Patients who kneel frequently such as carpet fitters are very prone to developing prepatellar bursitis.

Examination focusing on a swelling

The affected area or joint should be examined and also the local lymph nodes.

The following points relate to a swelling or mass rather than a joint effusion, which should be obvious on clinical examination.

When examining a lump or swelling the following points should be elicited.

Site
Which limb is affected and where is the lesion?

Skin
- Is the lesion within the skin, in the subcutaneous tissue or deep to the fascia? Painful deep lesions are suspicious and need investigation.
- Is the skin normal over the lesion, inflamed or abnormal?

Consistency

Is the lesion soft, firm or hard? A lipoma is often described as firm.

Diffuse or discrete

Some swellings are large without clear margins and appear to merge with the surrounding structures, whereas others are more easily palpable.

Surface

Is the surface of the lesion smooth or irregular?

Mobile or fixed

A discrete mass may be fixed to the underlying structures, like a ganglion, or more mobile, e.g. a lipoma.

Fluctuance

Fluctuant lesions contain fluid, such as a Baker's cyst.

Pulsatile

Pulsatile and expansile lesions are vascular aneurysms.

Transillumination

Fluid-filled or soft lesions (e.g. lipoma) will transilluminate when tested with a pen torch if the fluid is clear.

The patient presenting with joint swelling only

This has been covered in Chapters 2 and 3. Occasionally a patient will present with swelling of a single large joint and this can be the onset of a generalized condition such as rheumatoid arthritis.

Therefore examine other joints such as the hand (if rheumatoid arthritis is suspected) or the spine (if ankylosing spondylitis).

Investigation of a patient with a swelling

We will consider joint swelling as a separate condition from a discrete swelling or mass.

Joint swelling (effusion)

Exclude infection (see Ch. 3).

Blood tests should be carried out, including rheumatoid factor and autoantibodies to look for inflammatory arthritis.

X-rays may show osteoarthritis/rheumatoid arthritis or be normal.

Synovial fluid analysis is performed for gout and pseudogout.

A limb swelling or lump

Further investigation may be unnecessary.

For example, a patient has a cystic lesion on the volar aspect of the wrist, which comes and goes and is fixed to deep structures. The lesion is firm, smooth and transilluminates. This patient has a ganglion and this can be confirmed by aspirating jelly-like fluid.

Further investigation is necessary if there is doubt about a diagnosis.

- If bony pathology is suspected an X-ray of the affected limb should be performed. A benign or malignant bony lesion may be found.
- A deeply situated soft tissue lesion may be a sarcoma and if so needs further investigation.

An initial ultrasound scan may be useful to confirm the presence of a mass and whether it is fluid filled or solid.

However, an MRI scan with contrast gives detail regarding the exact nature of the lesion.

If doubt still exists, the patient should be referred to a specialist sarcoma service and the next step would be a biopsy.

An algorithm for the investigation of a limb swelling is given in Figure 6.1.

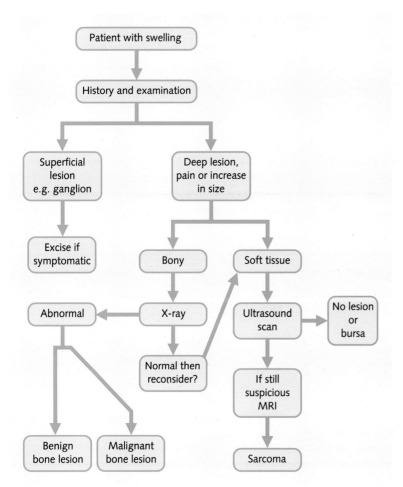

Fig. 6.1 Algorithm for the investigation of a limb swelling. MRI, magnetic resonance imaging.

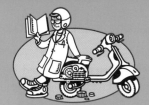

It is quite common for patients to present with bony lesions on X-ray. These are usually incidental findings (the X-ray was taken for another reason such as minor trauma and an abnormality is found) and cause great concern to patients.

Examples include a chest X-ray taken for respiratory disease showing a lesion in the clavicle or a pelvic X-ray taken for hip disease showing metastatic prostate carcinoma.

Differential diagnosis of a lesion on X-ray

Benign lesions are quite common.

Primary bone malignancy is extremely rare.

Secondary bone tumours are common in the elderly.

Infection can present as a bone lesion.

Benign tumours/disorders

- Osteochondroma.
- Osteoid osteoma.
- Enchondroma.
- Bone cysts.
- Fibrous dysplasia.

Malignant tumours

- Primary.
  —Osteosarcoma
  —Ewing's sarcoma
  —Chondrosarcoma
- Secondary—metastatic deposit:
  —Breast
  —Lung
  —Prostate
  —Renal
  —Thyroid
  —Bowel
- Haemopoietic diseases.
  —Myeloma
  —Lymphoma

Infection

- Osteomyelitis.

Metabolic bone disease

- Paget's disease.

Describing bone lesions on X-ray

 Practise describing bone defects and lesions whenever possible.

1. Name and age of patient.
2. Site—which bone and where in the bone:
   - The lesion can be in the diaphysis (shaft), metaphysis (cancellous bone between the growth plate and shaft) or epiphysis (between the growth plate and the joint).
   - The lesion can primarily affect either the cortex or medulla of the bone.
3. Appearance:
   - The lesion can be lytic (e.g. breast metastasis) (Fig. 7.1), sclerotic (e.g. prostate metastasis), mixed or calcified (enchondroma).

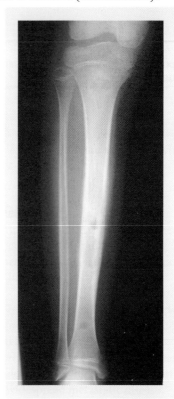

Fig. 7.1 Lytic lesion suggestive of malignancy.

Past medical history

 A previous history of carcinoma is extremely important when dealing with such a patient. The lesion should be treated as a metastatic lesion until proven otherwise.

Breast malignancy can be dormant for many years prior to re-presenting with metastases.

Examination focusing on a patient with an X-ray abnormality
Site
Different lesions are more common in certain locations, for example enchondromas are more common in the hand.

Secondary bone metastases tend to be found in the central skeleton.

Limb examination
Examination of the affected limb will usually be normal.

Tenderness, redness and swelling would be present in:
- Impending or actual fracture associated with a bone metastasis.
- Osteomyelitis.
- Osteoid osteoma.
- Malignant primary bone tumour.

Malignant secondaries or bone lesions from haemopoietic diseases rarely show any external features.

Generalized
In secondary malignancy with unknown primary, it is important to examine:
- Breast (for carcinoma).
- Chest (for lung tumours).
- Abdomen (for renal or bowel tumours and evidence of haemopoietic disease such as liver and spleen enlargement).
- Per rectum (PR) (prostate).
- Thyroid (for carcinoma).

Investigation of a bone lesion on X-ray
The X-ray
It is important to obtain two views taken at 90° to one another and to obtain full-length views of the entire bone (to ensure there are no further lesions along the same bone).

Most benign lesions need no further investigation and repeat X-rays after 6 months are useful to ensure the bone lesion does not change in appearance and develop any sinister features.

Further investigation
Further investigation is only necessary if there is doubt about the diagnosis or to confirm or exclude malignancy.

Blood tests
- A full blood count (FBC) may show anaemia of chronic disease.
- Liver function tests (LFTs) could be deranged if liver metastases are present.
- The calcium profile is often raised in generalized malignancy, and alkaline phosphatase is raised in Paget's disease.
- C-reactive protein (CRP) and erythrocyte sedimentation rate (ESR) are raised in infection or malignancy.
- A very high ESR suggests myeloma. It is confirmed with serum electrophoresis and urinary Bence Jones proteins.
- Prostate-specific antigen (PSA) is elevated in prostate malignancy.
- Carcinoembryonic antigen (CEA) is elevated in bowel carcinoma.

Isotope bone scan
This is a very useful tool to detect further lesions in malignancy or to see if a lesion is active (i.e. hot on bone scan). Infection will show up 'hot' as will malignant lesions.

Of the benign lesions only osteoid osteoma will show increased uptake.

Computed tomography (CT)
CT is used to confirm osteoid osteoma.

Magnetic resonance imaging (MRI)
MRI can detect early metastatic lesions before X-ray features are apparent.

It is also used to define the extent of malignant bone tumours and can help to distinguish between benign and malignant lesions.

Biopsy

It can be very difficult to be certain of the diagnosis in some cases. A biopsy will prove whether the tumour is benign or malignant and exclude infection as the cause.

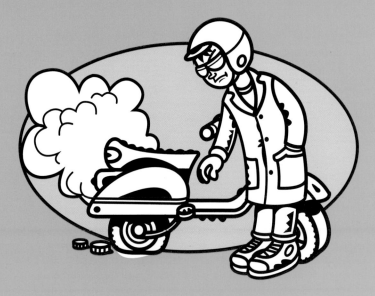

DISEASES AND DISORDERS

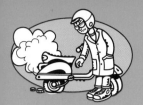

8. Osteoarthritis

Definition

Osteoarthritis (OA) is a non-inflammatory disorder of synovial joints characterized by articular surface wear and formation of new bone (attempts at repair). It is also known as degenerative joint disease and characterized by joint pain, stiffness and swelling of joints.

Incidence

Osteoarthritis is the most common joint disease, affecting up to 85% of the population at some time in their lives. It is often asymptomatic and the true prevalence of symptomatic OA in the western world is around 20%.

Pathology and aetiology

Histologically the weight-bearing cartilage surface degenerates and eventually wears away completely, exposing the subchondral bone, which becomes eburnated (Fig. 8.1). Cysts occur because of microfracture of the articular surface and new bone laid down (sclerosis) in the surrounding bone. Disorganized new bone is produced at the margins of joints (osteophytes) as the disease progresses. In addition to this, the synovial lining becomes thickened and inflamed, often producing excess synovial fluid (an effusion).

 These changes explain the four cardinal features seen on X-ray of joint space: narrowing, sclerosis, cysts and osteophytes.

Osteoarthritis is described as primary where no underlying cause is found or secondary where there is a clear predisposing factor.

Primary osteoarthritis has many aetiological factors but the exact cause is not known. A variety of genetic and environmental factors are implicated in causing osteoarthritis. This type of arthritis is more common in women and increases with age.

In secondary osteoarthritis a cause is clearly identified and these are shown in Figure 8.2.

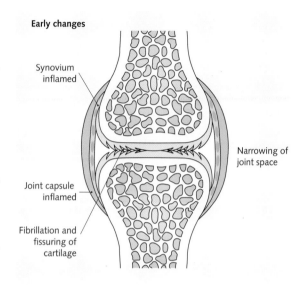

Early changes

- Synovium inflamed
- Narrowing of joint space
- Joint capsule inflamed
- Fibrillation and fissuring of cartilage

Changes secondary to loss of cartilage

- (Outgrowth of bone) osteophytes
- Hyperplasia of synovium
- Subarticular cyst
- Thickening and eburnation of bone

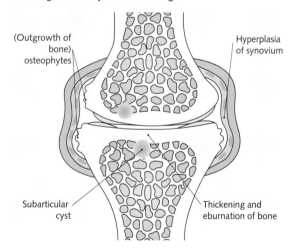

Fig. 8.1 Pathological changes in osteoarthritis.

Clinical features

The presenting complaints of patients with osteoarthritis are variable. The patient is usually systemically well and complains of pain which is usually aching or burning in nature and localized to the joint but may be referred to the joint below.

The history is usually of gradually increasing, asymmetrical joint pain over several years, the level

Secondary causes of osteoarthritis

Congenital/developmental

Developmental dysplasia of the hip
Perthes disease
Slipped upper femoral epiphysis

Acquired
Trauma:
• Fractures involving joint surfaces
• Fractures causing significant deformity
• Ligamentous injury causing joint instability
Infection—septic arthritis
Avascular necrosis
Inflammatory arthritis, e.g. rheumatoid arthritis
Neuropathic—Charcot joints
Metabolic, e.g. Paget's disease
Iatrogenic—post-surgery, e.g. meniscectomy

Fig. 8.2 Secondary causes of osteoarthritis.

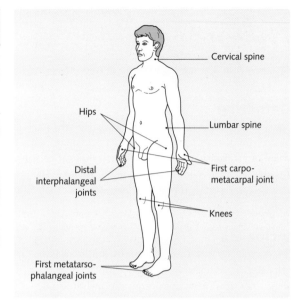

Fig. 8.3 Joints commonly affected by osteoarthritis.

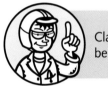 Classically pain in the hip can be referred to the knee.

of which is variable but can be severe. The pain is worse after activity and relieved by rest, and as the disease progresses night pain can be a feature. Occasionally patients present with rapidly destructive OA, which can mimic a septic or inflammatory arthritis.

Patients can present with only one or multiple joint involvement.

Other symptoms include swelling, deformity (bow legs—varus knee), stiffness and weakness (usually secondary to wasting). Patients will also complain they are unable to do certain activities, which may be recreational or more basic activities of daily living (for example, patients with severe osteoarthritis of the hip are unable to put on socks or cut their own toenails).

Almost any synovial joint can be affected by osteoarthritis, most commonly the knee, hip, hands (often the first carpometacarpal joint), fingers (distal interphalangeal (DIP) joints) but also the spine, shoulder, elbow and wrist (Figs 8.3 and 8.4).

The examination begins as the patient enters the room.

• Look for a limp, use of a stick and how reliant the patient is on relatives for simple tasks such as undressing for examination.

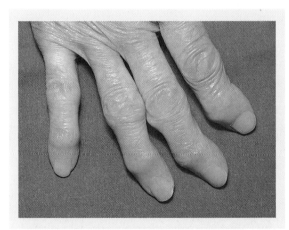

Fig. 8.4 Osteoarthritis of the hand, showing Herberden's nodes at the distal interphalangeal joints and Bouchard's nodes at the proximal interphalangeal joints (from Haslett C, Chilvers E R, Boon N A et al (eds) 2002 Davidson's principles and practice of medicine, 19th edn. Churchill Livingstone, Edinburgh).

• Deformity may be obvious but also note previous scars, redness, swelling and wasting of muscles on inspection.
• Palpate for an effusion, joint line tenderness and crepitus (cracking noise can be heard in severe cases).
• The range of movement of the particular joint will be diminished and there may be fixed deformity.
• The joints above and below should be examined.

Classic features of osteoarthritis include Herberden's nodes of the DIP joint and a Baker's cyst behind the knee.

Diagnosis and Investigation

In many cases the diagnosis is clear from the history and clinical examination, and apart from a plain X-ray further investigation may be unnecessary.

Blood tests may be required to exclude septic or inflammatory arthritis in atypical cases if the treating doctor is not certain of the diagnosis.

X-rays will usually show decreased joint space, sclerosis, subchondral cysts and osteophytes (Fig. 8.5).

Management

There is no cure for osteoarthritis and treatment is aimed at relieving pain and maintaining function. The treatment for osteoarthritis can be conservative or surgical.

Conservative

- Initially lifestyle advice including weight loss, regular exercise and avoidance of impact loading activities is given. Non-steroidal anti-inflammatory drugs such as diclofenac are good in the early stages providing the patient does not have a history of peptic ulceration. Other regular analgesia such as codeine and paracetamol should be prescribed if required.
- Physiotherapy improves gait and function of an affected limb, and simple measures such as a walking stick reduce pain on walking.
- Glucosamine is widely taken by the population at large and has a small beneficial effect.
- Injections of corticosteroids are useful for temporary relief, especially in patients unfit for surgery; however, there is a small risk of infection. New treatments such as hyaluronic acid derivatives given by injection are expensive and not yet proven.

Surgical

Surgical treatments for osteoarthritis depend on the age of the patient, the joint involved and the level of pain and disability experienced. This is dealt with in more detail in Chapter 18.

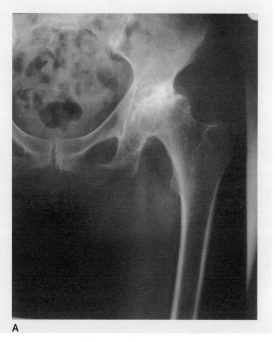

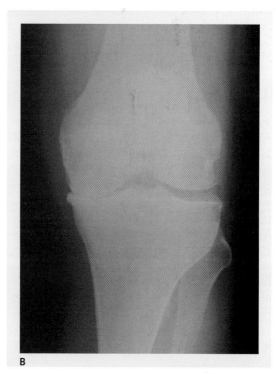

Fig. 8.5 Features of osteoarthritis on X-ray: (A) hip; (B) knee.

The decision to operate can be difficult to make, as all surgery has risks and complications. Surgery may help when the patient says, 'I cannot cope any longer with the pain.'

There are five things a surgeon can do to a joint:

1. Debride and washout. This is usually done for osteoarthritis of the knee and gives temporary relief in some patients.
2. Joint replacement. This is most commonly of the hip or knee. It gives excellent pain relief in 90% of patients for at least 10 years.
3. Joint fusion. The two sides are removed and fused together. This is most commonly used around the foot and ankle; good pain relief is achieved provided fusion occurs but obviously movement is lost.
4. Joint excision. This is less commonly used nowadays. It is still used occasionally in the first metatarsophalangeal (MTP) joint and where other methods have failed (e.g. hip—Girdlestone's procedure).
5. Realignment surgery. Increased load passing through a joint because of a deformity often leads to osteoarthritis. The surgeon can realign the limb by breaking the bone above or below the joint, removing a wedge of bone and correcting the deformity. The most common site for this procedure is the knee. The patient will usually have a varus deformity of the knee (bow legs). The tibia is realigned to redistribute the load more evenly, slowing the progression of osteoarthritis. See Figure 8.6.

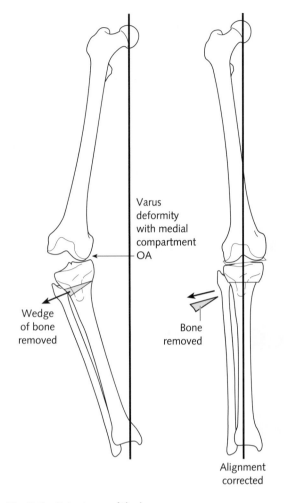

Fig. 8.6 Osteotomy of the knee.

- How common is osteoarthritis?
- How do you classify osteoarthritis?
- What causes of secondary osteoarthritis are there?
- Outline the pathological process involved in the development of osteoarthritis.
- Define osteoarthritis. What is it also known as?
- What symptoms do patients complain of?
- Which joints are commonly affected by osteoarthritis?
- On examination what physical signs are present?
- What are the X-ray features of osteoarthritis?
- What treatment options are available?
- If surgery is necessary what types of operations are available?

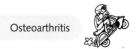

Further reading

Dandy D J 1998 Essentials of orthopaedics and trauma, 3rd edn. Churchill Livingstone, London

Fitzgerald R H, Kaufer H, Malkani A (eds) 2002 Orthopaedics. Mosby, Philadelphia

Miller M D 2000 Review of orthopaedics, 3rd edn. WB Saunders, Philadelphia

Solomon L, Warwick D, Nayagan D (eds) 2001 Apley's system of orthopaedics and fractures, 8th edn. Hodder Arnold, London

Orthoteers website: http://www.orthoteers.co.uk

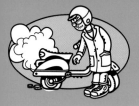

9. Rheumatoid Arthritis

Definition

Rheumatoid arthritis (RA) is a common inflammatory condition. It is characterized by arthritis that is usually polyarticular and follows a chronic course, resulting in significant disability. RA is a systemic disease and is associated with a reduction in life expectancy. Other systems may also be involved.

 RA has a major impact on patients' lives. After 20 years, 80% of patients are disabled. Life expectancy is reduced by between 3 and 18 years.

Incidence and prevalence

RA affects females more commonly than males. Most studies show a female-to-male excess of between two and four times. The annual incidence in the UK is 0.1–0.2/1000 in males and 0.2–0.4/1000 in females. RA prevalence in Europeans and North American Caucasians is close to 1%.

Aetiology

The aetiology of RA has not been explained. It appears to be multifactorial, with both genetic and environmental factors having an important influence.

Genetic factors

Genetic factors contribute approximately 50% to the aetiology. The inheritance of certain human leucocyte antigen (HLA) genes explains about 30% of the total genetic effect. HLA-DR4 is particularly important. Several subtypes of the DR4 gene increase RA susceptibility and severity.

Environmental factors

Environmental influences on the development of RA are not well understood. People have examined the effects of various infections, occupations and lifestyle factors, but no links have been found.

Immunological abnormalities

In rheumatoid arthritis, the immunological mechanisms that usually protect the body by fighting infections and destroying malignant cells target normal tissue, resulting in joint damage. T-lymphocytes play a key role in the initiation of inflammation in RA Figs 9.1–9.3).

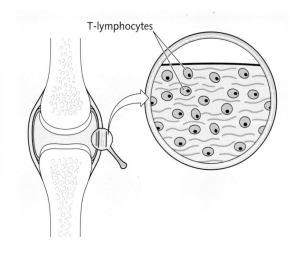

Fig. 9.1 T-lymphocytes (predominantly T-helper cells) accumulate in the synovium.

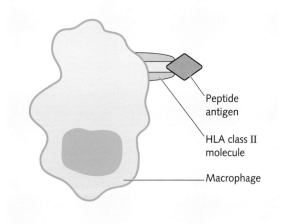

Fig. 9.2 Synovial macrophages (antigen-presenting cells) express peptide antigens on their cell surfaces in association with human lymphocyte antigen (HLA) class 2 molecules.

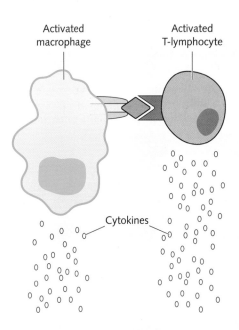

Fig. 9.3 T-lymphocytes with appropriate receptors interact with the macrophages and both cell types become activated.

The activated cells produce cytokines (intercellular messenger proteins), e.g. tumour necrosis factor-α (TNF-α), interleukin-1 (IL-1). These cytokines have many actions, including those shown in Figure 9.4.

Rheumatoid factor is found in the serum of approximately 80% of patients with RA. High levels are associated with more severe disease and the presence of extra-articular features.

Pathology

The main pathological abnormality in RA is synovitis. As inflammatory cells infiltrate the synovium, it proliferates. Chronically inflamed tissue (pannus)

Actions of cytokines
Stimulation of inflammation
Attraction of other immune cells
Excess synovial fluid production
Cartilage destruction
Bone resorption
Stimulation of B-lymphocyte differentiation and maturation
Increased antibody production, including production of Rheumatoid factor

Fig. 9.4 Actions of cytokines.

extends from the joint margins, and erodes the articular cartilage (Fig. 9.5). Extensive erosion of cartilage and bone, with concomitant involvement of ligaments and joint capsules, leads to joint deformity.

Subcutaneous rheumatoid nodules are found in up to 20% of patients. They usually accompany severe disease and are possibly due to small vessel vasculitis. Histology reveals a central area of fibrinoid necrosis surrounded by fibroblasts.

Clinical features

RA can develop at any time of life from infancy to old age. The peak age of onset is in the fourth and fifth decades. Symptoms usually begin gradually, developing over weeks or months. However, some people experience an acute onset and are able to remember the exact date that they first felt unwell.

The clinical features of RA can be divided into:
- Articular features.
- Extra-articular features.
  - systemic
  - periarticular
  - affecting distant organs.

Articular features of RA

The usual presenting symptoms of rheumatoid arthritis are joint pain, stiffness and swelling. These are classically symmetrical, affecting the wrists and small joints of the hands and feet, but may follow different patterns.

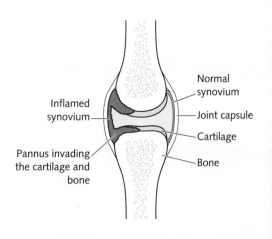

Fig. 9.5 Diagram of a synovial joint. One side is healthy, the other shows the pathological changes of RA.

Monoarthritis

Occasionally, a patient presents with a monoarthritis of a larger joint such as the knee or shoulder.

Palindromic rheumatism

Synovitis appears to move rapidly from one region to another (Fig. 9.6). Inflammation of one or more joints begins acutely, lasts for hours or days and then settles quickly. Patients experience recurrent attacks and many go on to develop typical RA.

Joint stiffness is usually noticed on waking in the morning and tends to improve as the day progresses. The duration of this early-morning stiffness is a useful marker of disease activity.

Pain and stiffness lead to varying degrees of functional loss. Even in the early stages of the disease, patients can struggle with everyday tasks such as dressing and turning on taps because of active synovitis. In established RA, joint destruction results in further limitations.

Synovitis causes 'boggy' joint swelling. The skin overlying an affected joint is usually warm and red due to increased local blood flow. On palpation, the swelling is tender and has a similar consistency to that of a grape.

The effects of RA on specific joint regions

The rheumatoid hand and wrist The hands and wrists are almost always involved in RA (Fig. 9.7). Synovitis typically occurs in the wrists, metacarpophalangeal (MCP) and proximal interphalangeal (PIP) joints, sparing the distal interphalangeal (DIP) joints. This inflammation can weaken the ligaments and tendons, producing well-recognized deformities.

Ulnar deviation of the fingers results from metacarpophalangeal joint synovitis (Fig. 9.8). Subluxation of the metacarpophalangeal joints can occur, with the proximal phalanges drifting in an ulnar and volar direction.

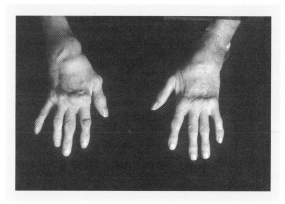

Fig. 9.7 The hands of a patient with RA. Note the synovitis of the wrists, metacarpophalangeal and proximal interphalangeal joints.

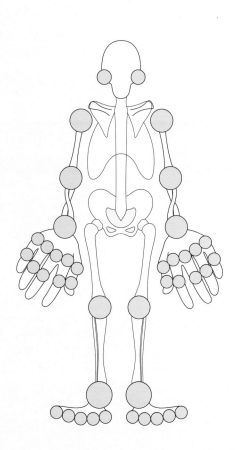

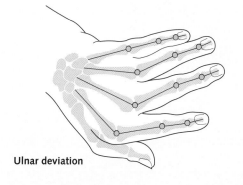

Ulnar deviation

Fig. 9.6 The joints most commonly affected by RA.

Fig. 9.8 Ulnar deviation.

Boutonnière and swan-neck deformities of the digits are due to proximal interphalangeal joint synovitis and laxity and/or contractures of the extensor and flexor apparatus (Fig. 9.9). The boutonnière deformity is characterized by PIP flexion and DIP hyperextension. With swan-neck deformity there is MCP flexion, PIP hyperextension and DIP flexion.

Radial deviation of the wrist occurs to compensate partly for ulnar deviation of the fingers. Subluxation of the wrist results in prominence of the ulnar styloid.

The foot Forefoot synovitis is common in rheumatoid arthritis. The proximal phalanges sublux

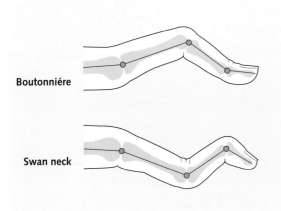

Fig. 9.9 Boutonnière and swan-neck deformities.

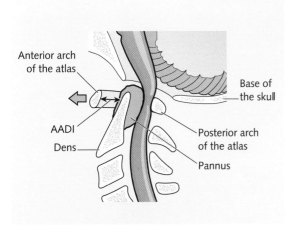

Fig. 9.10 In normal adults, the distance between the anterior arch of the atlas and the dens (anterior atlanto-dental interspace, or AADI) should not exceed 3 mm. The diagram shows forward subluxation of the atlas on the axis. The spinal cord is compressed between pannus around the dens and the posterior arch of the atlas.

dorsally and the metatarsal heads become eroded and displaced towards the floor. They can be easily palpated through the sole of the foot and make weight bearing very uncomfortable. Patients often feel as though they are 'walking on marbles'. Hindfoot involvement can also cause problems, with subtalar arthritis. Patients with established disease develop valgus deformities here with collapse of the longitudinal arch.

The cervical spine It is important to recognize involvement of the cervical spine in RA. Inflammation and erosive disease, affecting the uncovertebral joints and stabilizing ligaments of the first two cervical vertebrae, can result in atlantoaxial subluxation. The atlas slips forward on the axis, reducing the space around the spinal cord (Fig. 9.10). This produces neck pain that radiates to the occiput. Upper motor neuron damage resulting in a spastic quadriparesis is a rare complication.

Damage to the articulation between the occiput and atlas may allow the odontoid peg to move upwards, through the foramen magnum. This can threaten the cervical cord and brainstem, sometimes resulting in sudden death after minor jolts to the head and neck.

It is important to take lateral flexion X-rays of the cervical spine in RA patients requiring a general anaesthetic. The anaesthetist must be aware of any cervical instability so that precautions can be taken during intubation.

Extra-articular features of RA
Periarticular features
In addition to joint inflammation, patients with RA often experience other musculoskeletal problems.

Rheumatoid nodules Rheumatoid nodules are firm subcutaneous swellings that tend to develop in areas affected by pressure or friction, such as the fingers, elbows and Achilles tendon. They are seen in patients who test positive for rheumatoid factor. Nodulosis at any site can be complicated by infection.

Tenosynovitis and bursitis Tendon sheaths and bursae are lined with synovium. This can become inflamed in RA, resulting in tenosynovitis and bursitis. The flexor tendons of the fingers are often affected by tenosynovitis. Pain is felt in the palm of the hand and volar aspect of the wrist. Active flexion of the fingers is reduced, whilst passive movements remain full. Both flexion and extension are painful and may be accompanied by crepitus. Flexor tenosynovitis in the carpal tunnel can compress the median nerve. The olecranon and subacromial bursae are common sites of bursitis.

Carpal tunnel syndrome Synovitis can cause entrapment of peripheral nerves. Median nerve compression resulting in carpal tunnel syndrome is common.

Systemic features of RA

As well as causing joint pain and swelling, active RA makes people feel generally unwell. The inflammation can result in systemic symptoms such as fever, weight loss and lethargy. These can be prominent, particularly in people with acute-onset RA, in whom infection and malignancy are important differential diagnoses.

The effects of RA on distant organs

RA can affect many body systems (Fig. 9.11). Extra-articular disease can be serious and is associated with an increase in mortality.

Anaemia Anaemia of RA can be due to:
- Anaemia of chronic disease.
- Autoimmune haemolysis.
- Felty's syndrome.

Drugs used in the treatment of RA can also induce anaemia. Non-steroidal anti-inflammatory drugs can cause iron deficiency as a result of chronic blood loss from gastrointestinal inflammation. Disease-modifying antirheumatic drugs sometimes produce anaemia via bone marrow suppression.

Felty's syndrome Felty's syndrome is the association of RA with splenomegaly and leucopenia. It usually occurs in patients who are rheumatoid factor positive. The leucopenia leads to frequent bacterial infections. Lymphadenopathy, anaemia and thrombocytopenia can also occur.

Rheumatoid lung disease Although pulmonary disease is common in RA, it does not always produce

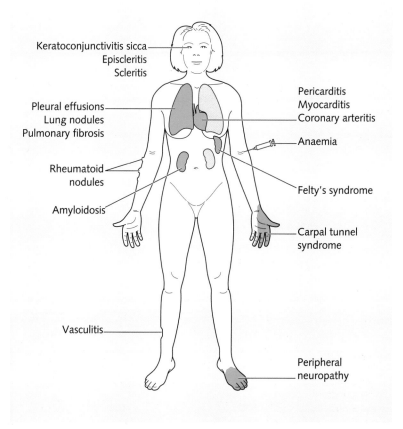

Fig. 9.11 Extra-articular manifestations of RA.

Keratoconjunctivitis sicca
Episcleritis
Scleritis

Pleural effusions
Lung nodules
Pulmonary fibrosis

Rheumatoid nodules

Amyloidosis

Vasculitis

Pericarditis
Myocarditis
Coronary arteritis

Anaemia

Felty's syndrome

Carpal tunnel syndrome

Peripheral neuropathy

symptoms. Males are more frequently affected than females.

Pleural effusions can occur early in the disease, sometimes preceding the arthritis. Rheumatoid factor can be detected in the fluid, which is a transudate.

Lung nodules are found in patients who are seropositive and usually have subcutaneous nodules. They rarely cause symptoms, but can cavitate or become infected.

Pneumonitis can lead to pulmonary fibrosis.

Cardiac disease Like lung disease, pericardial inflammation is common in RA, but rarely symptomatic. Pericardial effusions can occur. Myocarditis is a rare manifestation of RA. Coronary arteritis is also rare and usually occurs as part of a generalized vasculitis.

Eye disease Keratoconjunctivitis sicca affects at least 10% of patients with RA. Eyes are dry because of reduced tear production and the cornea and conjunctiva can become damaged. Episcleritis and scleritis are less common. Both cause redness and often pain of the eye. Severe scleritis can rarely result in spontaneous scleral perforation, so needs treating aggressively.

Amyloidosis Secondary amyloidosis develops as a result of chronic inflammation. Many organs can be infiltrated, including the kidneys, heart, liver and gastrointestinal tract. Proteinuria due to renal disease is the commonest manifestation of amyloidosis in RA. Prognosis is poor.

Vasculitis Vasculitis occasionally complicates RA. It predominates in patients who are seropositive for rheumatoid factor and have severe disease. Common clinical features include leg ulcers and peripheral neuropathy. Rarely, there is involvement of coronary or cerebral vessels which leads to cardiac or cerebral ischaemia.

Investigations

RA should be considered in all patients presenting with joint inflammation, irrespective of the number or distribution of involved joints.

The following investigations are useful:

Blood tests

Full blood count may show anaemia of chronic disease, thrombocytosis secondary to inflammation or leucopenia of Felty's syndrome.

Erythrocyte sedimentation rate, C-reactive protein or plasma viscosity is usually raised in the presence of synovitis and they are useful markers of response to treatment.

Rheumatoid factor is found in the serum of 70–90% of RA patients, but is often not detectable during the first few months of the disease. Those patients who lack the antibodies are sometimes described as having 'seronegative rheumatoid arthritis'. It is important to remember that rheumatoid factor is also found in at least 1% of the normal population.

A diagnosis of RA should not be made purely on the presence of a positive rheumatoid factor and should not be excluded because rheumatoid factor is absent.

Radiological investigations

Plain X-rays should be obtained to look for signs of RA (Fig. 9.12). These tend to be seen first in the small joints of the hands and feet (Figs 9.13 and 9.14).

Radiological changes are often not apparent when patients first present with RA. In patients with normal X-rays, but persistent symptoms, it is useful to repeat the X-rays after several months. Erosions can be detected sooner using ultrasound or magnetic resonance imaging.

The tests discussed above are always useful in the investigation of patients with possible RA. However, different clinical presentations often require additional investigations.

The four main radiological signs of RA
Soft tissue swelling Periarticular osteoporosis Juxta-articular erosions Narrowing of joint space

Fig. 9.12 The four main radiological signs of RA.

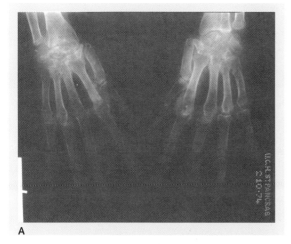

A

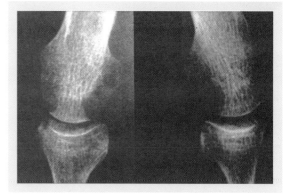

Fig. 9.14 Large erosions of two MCP joints.

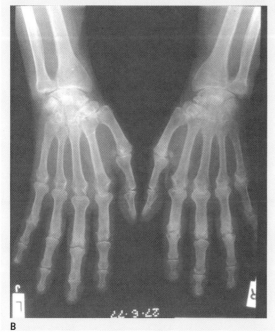

B

Fig. 9.13 Both radiographs show periarticular osteopaenia and erosions of the MCP and PIP joints. The carpal bones are severely eroded in Fig. 9.13A.

Management

Patients with RA should be cared for by a multidisciplinary team. Figure 18.8 (p. 131) lists the operations commonly performed on patients with RA. Figure 9.15 lists the professionals involved in the care of RA patients and gives details of the roles they play.

Drug treatment

There are two main aims of drug treatment in RA:
- Reduction of symptoms.
- Prevention of damage by control of disease.

Non-steroidal anti-inflammatory drugs (NSAIDs)

NSAIDs can improve joint pain and stiffness, but have no effect on disease activity or progression. If a patient does not respond to one NSAID, it is worth substituting another.

Corticosteroids

Corticosteroids can swiftly improve pain and swelling in RA. Low doses of oral prednisolone are often used to control symptoms early in the disease before DMARDs (see below) become effective. Corticosteroids can be given intra-articularly to treat local synovitis and are sometimes given via the intramuscular or intravenous route for a generalized flare of rheumatoid arthritis.

Disease-modifying antirheumatic drugs (DMARDs)

DMARDs are capable of suppressing disease activity and may slow progression of erosive joint damage. Some DMARDs suppress the immune system; others inhibit cell replication. However, for many of these drugs, the mechanism of action is not completely understood.

DMARDs are usually prescribed soon after the diagnosis of RA is made. They are slow-acting and take weeks or months to produce a clinical effect. If a patient does not respond adequately to one DMARD, a second can be added or substituted. Three or more DMARDs may be required to have an impact on severe RA.

Like many drugs, DMARDs can cause minor side-effects, including nausea, headache and rashes (Fig. 9.16). More serious complications such as bone

Fig. 9.15 Professionals involved in the care of RA patients and the roles they play.

Professionals involved in the care of RA patients and the roles they play	
Professional	**Role**
Rheumatologist	Monitoring of disease activity Prescription and monitoring of drug therapy Identification and management of complications Referral to other specialists when necessary Coordination of team
Orthopaedic surgeon	Replacement of damaged joints Surgical synovectomy
Physiotherapist	Use of physical therapies to combat inflammation (e.g. ice, warmth) Prescription of exercises to maintain and improve muscular strength and range of joint movement
Occupational therapist	Splinting of acutely inflamed joints Advice on how to function whilst putting as little stress as possible on the joints (joint protection) Provision of aids and appliances to assist with activities of daily living
Podiatrist	Assessment of footwear and advice on choosing suitable shoes Provision of insoles to improve the mechanics of deformed feet Prevention and treatment of skin lesions, such as calluses and ulcers

Fig. 9.16 Some disease-modifying drugs and their potential side-effects.

Some disease-modifying drugs and their potential side-effects	
DMARD	**Possible side-effects**
Azathioprine	Gastrointestinal (GI) upset Bone marrow suppression
Cyclophosphamide	Bone marrow suppression Increased risk of malignancy Infertility
Ciclosporin	Renal impairment Hypertension Bone marrow suppression
Gold	Rash Proteinuria Bone marrow suppression
Hydroxychloroquine	Retinal damage
Leflunomide	Hypertension GI upset Bone marrow suppression
Methotrexate	GI upset Oral ulcers Raised liver enzymes Pneumonitis Bone marrow suppression
D-penicillamine	Rash Proteinuria Bone marrow suppression
Sulfasalazine	GI upset Raised liver enzymes Bone marrow suppression

marrow suppression, abnormal liver function and renal impairment are rarer, but well recognized. It is therefore important to monitor patients receiving DMARD therapy. The monitoring protocol depends on the drug prescribed. For example, a patient taking methotrexate should have a full blood count and tests of liver and renal function performed at intervals of 4–8 weeks.

Biological therapies
Biological therapies that target inflammatory mediators in RA have recently been introduced. Etanercept, a soluble TNF-α receptor, and infliximab, a monoclonal antibody against TNF-α, are proving to be very effective. Drugs that manipulate other cytokines are in various stages of development.

Although biological therapies are producing good clinical results, little is known about their long-term safety. In the short term, there is a worry that they might increase the risk of serious infection. These drugs are currently reserved for patients who have failed to respond to therapy with several DMARDs, but in the near future they may be used early in the disease.

- Which HLA type is associated with rheumatoid arthritis (RA)?
- What role do cytokines play in the pathogenesis of RA?
- What is pannus?
- Which joints are commonly affected by RA?
- What are the common deformities seen in the rheumatoid hand?
- What complications can occur when RA affects the cervical spine?
- List the four main radiological signs of RA.
- List the extra-articular manifestations of RA.
- List the causes of anaemia in RA.
- Discuss the role of members of the multidisciplinary team.
- Name some disease-modifying antirheumatic drugs (DMARDs) used in the treatment of RA.

Further reading
Cooper N J 2000 Economic burden of rheumatoid arthritis: a systematic review. *Rheumatology* **39**: 28–33

Emery P, Moreland L W 2003 *TNF inhibition in the treatment of rheumatoid arthritis*. Taylor & Francis

Gordon D A and Hastings D E 2003 Clinical features of rheumatoid arthritis. In: Hochberg et al (eds) *Rheumatology*, 3rd edn. Mosby, London, p 765–780

O'Dell J R 2001 Combinations of conventional disease modifying anti-rheumatic drugs. *Rheum Dis Clin North Am* **27**: 415–26

10. Spondyloarthropathies

Definition

The term 'spondyloarthropathy' (SPA) (or 'spondyloarthritis') describes a group of related and often overlapping inflammatory joint disorders (Fig. 10.1). The SPAs are distinct from rheumatoid arthritis. They are characterized by enthesitis as well as synovitis, and occur in patients who are seronegative for rheumatoid factor. For this reason, they are sometimes referred to as 'seronegative spondyloarthropathies'.

An enthesis is the insertion of a tendon, ligament or capsule into bone.

Aetiology

All types of SPA are genetically associated with HLA-B27, a major histocompatibility complex (MHC) class 1 antigen. HLA-B27 is more closely linked with some SPAs than others. It is most prevalent in ankylosing spondylitis, affecting 85–95% of these patients. The antigen is carried by approximately 10% of healthy Caucasians.

The true aetiology of the SPAs is unknown. Infection is thought to be important.

Bacterial DNA and proteins have been detected in joints affected by reactive arthritis (see below) and it is thought that infection may play a role in the development of other SPAs. It is possible that bacteria trigger an immune reaction in genetically predisposed people. There is an association with inflammatory bowel disease, which may be explained by an increase in the permeability of the gut to pathogens.

Pathology

The entheses are the key sites of inflammation in SPA. Initial inflammation and erosion are followed by fibrosis and ossification, which can result in

ankylosis of joints. In ankylosing spondylitis (AS), the outer fibres of the vertebral discs become inflamed where they attach to the corners of the vertebral bodies. Erosions cause squaring of the vertebrae, and ossification leads to formation of syndesmophytes (bony bridges). The sacroiliac joints are commonly affected and often become fused. Synovitis is another feature of the SPAs. Peripheral joints tend to be more commonly involved in psoriatic and reactive arthritis than in enteropathic arthritis and AS.

Pathological changes are not always confined to the musculoskeletal system. Cardiac and pulmonary abnormalities can occur.

Ankylosing spondylitis

Clinical features

The prevalence of ankylosing spondylitis (AS) amongst Caucasians is 0.5–1%. It is three times more common in men than in women and tends to be more severe in men. It usually develops in early adulthood, with the peak age of onset being in the mid-20s. Presentation after the age of 45 years is rare.

AS should always be considered in young people presenting with inflammatory-sounding back pain.

Clinical features can be divided into two groups:
- Musculoskeletal.
- Extraskeletal.

Musculoskeletal features

Most symptoms in AS are due to spinal and sacroiliac disease. The typical patient presents with a gradual onset of lower back pain and stiffness. Symptoms are worse early in the morning and after long periods of rest. They usually improve with exercise. Involvement of the thoracic spine and enthesitis at the costochondral junctions may cause chest pain.

The spondyloarthropathies
Ankylosing spondylitis
Psoriatic arthropathy
Reactive arthritis
Reiter's syndrome
Enteropathic arthritis

Fig. 10.1 The spondyloarthropathies.

Disease of the costovertebral joints can reduce chest expansion and restrict breathing.

In the early stages of the disease, patients may have few clinical signs. The sacroiliac joints are often tender and pain can be reproduced by applying physical stress to the joints. This can be achieved by applying pressure on the anterior superior iliac spines whilst the patient is lying supine.

Mobility of the lumbar spine is reduced. The Schober test is used to assess forward flexion in this region of the spine (see Fig. 10.2). With a pen, a mark is made on the skin at the lumbosacral joint, level with the dimples of Venus. A second mark is made 10 cm above. The patient bends forward with the legs straight and attempts to touch the floor. The distance between the two marks should increase by at least 5 cm.

 Some patients with AS have an abnormal Schober test, but are able to touch their toes because of good hip flexion.

Most patients with AS experience exacerbations and remissions. In those with severe disease, the spine becomes progressively stiffer and posture deteriorates (Fig. 10.3). The normal lumbar lordosis is lost and the thoracic and cervical spines become increasingly kyphotic. The resulting stooped posture further restricts chest expansion and causes the abdomen to protrude. It is sometimes referred to as the 'question-mark posture'. Spinal disease can be complicated by atlantoaxial subluxation and fractures.

The peripheral joints are involved less commonly than the axial skeleton in AS. Inflammation tends to target medium/large joints such as the shoulders, hips or knees. Pain and tenderness due to enthesitis can occur at many sites. Achilles tendonitis and plantar fasciitis are common examples of this.

Extraskeletal features
Systemic
Systemic features such as anorexia, fever, weight loss and fatigue trouble some patients, particularly early in the disease.

Acute anterior uveitis
Acute anterior uveitis (also called iritis) occurs in approximately one-third of patients with AS and does not correlate with the disease activity in the spine. The eye becomes red and painful and vision is blurred. It can be treated with steroid eye drops.

 Patients suffering from any spondyloarthropathy should be warned of the risk of uveitis and told to seek medical help if they develop a painful, red eye.

Cardiovascular disease
This occurs less frequently. Ascending aortitis, aortic incompetence and cardiac conduction disturbances tend to develop late in the disease.

Pulmonary fibrosis
Upper lobe pulmonary fibrosis is another late feature of AS.

Amyloidosis
This is a rare complication.

Fig. 10.2 The Schober test.

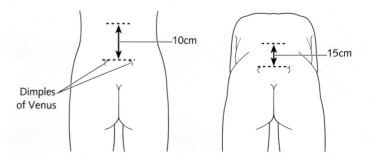

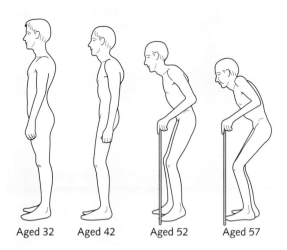

Fig. 10.3 Deterioration of posture in AS.

Investigations
Blood tests
A full blood count may reveal an anaemia of chronic disease.

Erythrocyte sedimentation rate (ESR) and C-reactive protein (CRP) are often raised during active phases of the disease.

Serological tests for rheumatoid factor are negative.

Genotyping for HLA-B27 is rarely requested. It is expensive and unnecessary for diagnosis, which can be made on clinical and radiological findings.

Radiological investigations
X-rays are the most useful investigations for AS. An anteroposterior view of the pelvis will show the sacroiliac joints. These appear normal initially, but later sclerosis and erosions are seen, sometimes progressing to complete fusion (Fig. 10.4). Views of the lumbar spine may show squaring of the vertebrae and formation of syndesmophytes (Fig 10.5). These are due to ossification of the longitudinal ligaments and produce a bamboo appearance. Radiographs taken at other sites of enthesitis may show erosions, for example at the insertion of the plantar fascia or Achilles tendon.

Management
Patients with AS should be cared for by a multidisciplinary team (see Ch. 9).

Physiotherapy
This is the most important element in the management of AS. Each patient should follow a

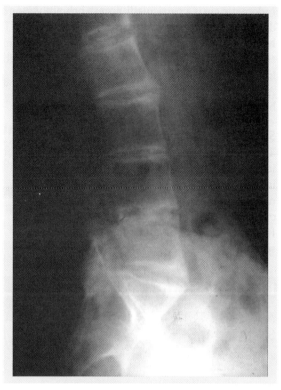

Fig. 10.4 Lateral radiograph showing syndesmophyte formation in the lumbar spine of a patient with advanced AS.

long-term exercise programme with the aim of maintaining normal posture and physical activity.

Drug treatment
Drug treatment can help to minimize pain and stiffness. Non-steroidal anti-inflammatory drugs (NSAIDs) should be used regularly, if tolerated.

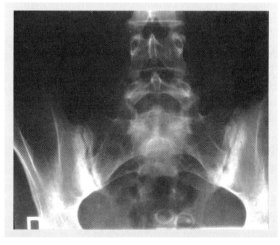

Fig. 10.5 Radiograph showing bilateral sacroiliitis.

Patterns of joint disease in psoriatic arthritis
Distal arthritis involving the distal interphalangeal (DIP) joints
Asymmetrical oligoarthritis
Symmetrical polyarthritis indistinguishable from rheumatoid arthritis (RA)
Spondylitis
Arthritis mutilans

Fig. 10.7 Patterns of joint disease in psoriatic arthritis.

extended to their original length. Psoriatic spondylitis tends to cause milder symptoms than classical AS, and sacroiliitis is often asymmetrical and asymptomatic. The uveitis and cardiac lesions seen in other SPAs can occur.

 Some patients present with articular features of psoriatic arthritis, but no history of skin disease. Careful inspection of areas such as the scalp and natal cleft may reveal small patches of psoriasis.

Investigations
Blood tests
Full blood count, ESR and CRP show a similar picture to that of AS.
Rheumatoid factor is usually absent.

Radiological investigations
The radiological changes of PsA are asymmetrical and target the small joints of the hands and feet,

Fig. 10.8 Psoriatic nail pitting.

particularly the DIP joints (Fig. 10.9). X-ray changes include:
- Erosions with proliferation of adjacent bone.
- Reabsorption of the terminal phalanges.
- Pencil-in-cup deformities.
- Periostitis.
- Ankylosis.
- New bone formation at entheses.

Sacroiliitis is found in up to 30% of cases and is usually asymmetrical.

Management
Peripheral joint arthritis and spinal disease in PsA are treated in the same way as in RA and AS respectively. Physiotherapy, NSAIDs and DMARD therapy are all commonly used.

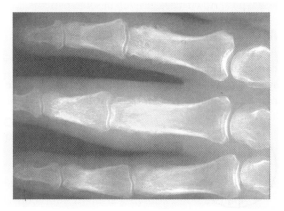

Fig. 10.9 Radiograph showing fluffy periosteal reaction and erosive changes in the digits of a patient with psoriatic arthritis.

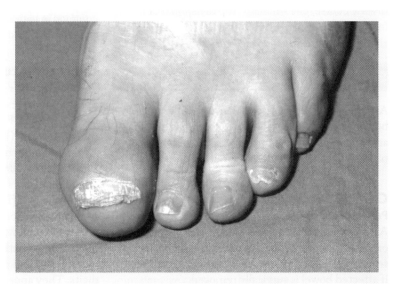

Prognosis

The prognosis of PsA is usually good. Joint function is well preserved in most cases, but in some, a chronic, progressive, deforming arthritis may develop.

- Which HLA type is associated with the spondyloarthropathies?
- Describe the pathological changes that affect the spine in ankylosing spondylitis.
- List the extraskeletal manifestations of ankylosing spondylitis.
- Describe the typical posture of a patient with ankylosing spondylitis.
- List some of the organisms known to trigger reactive arthritis.
- Apart from the joints, what other systems are affected by reactive arthritis?
- What triad of clinical features did Reiter describe?
- What are the five main patterns of joint disease in psoriatic arthritis?
- What are the radiological signs of psoriatic arthritis?

Further reading

Calin A, Taurog J D 1998 *The spondyloarthritides*. Oxford University Press, Oxford

Gladman D D 2002 Current concepts in psoriatic arthritis. *Curr Op Rheumatol* **14**: 361-366

Khan M A 1997 Spondyloarthropathies: Editorial review. *Curr Op Rheumatol* **9**: 281-283

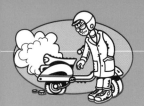

11. Connective Tissue Diseases

There is no strict definition of a connective tissue disease. The term is usually used to describe multisystem, inflammatory diseases that are associated with immunological abnormalities. There is overlap between these disorders, which share many clinical features (Fig. 11.1).

Systemic lupus erythematosus

Definition
Systemic lupus erythematosus (SLE) is an inflammatory disease that can involve almost any organ or system of the body.

Prevalence
SLE has a worldwide prevalence of 10–50 per 100,000. It affects women at least 10 times more frequently than it affects men, and is more common in Asian and Afro-Caribbean people than in Caucasians.

Aetiology
There are genetic, environmental and hormonal contributions to its aetiology. SLE can be induced by drugs, such as minocycline or hydralazine. Drug-induced lupus tends to be mild and settles when the offending drug is withdrawn.

Pathology
Immune function in SLE is abnormal, with abnormal cell-mediated immunity, B-cell hyperactivity and impaired immune complex clearance from tissues. A wide variety of autoantibodies have been described. The coagulation system may be abnormal and vasculopathy is frequent.

Clinical features
SLE usually develops between 15 and 40 years of age. The clinical features are diverse and the severity of the disease varies over time. Initial symptoms may be mild and rather vague, but it is the exacerbations of SLE and resultant tissue damage that cause significant ill-health. Severe lupus flares can result in life-threatening problems, including renal failure or cerebral vasculitis. Factors that may trigger flares of SLE are listed in Figure 11.2.

Non-specific features
Fatigue, malaise, fever and weight loss are common in SLE. The fatigue can be quite disabling and is difficult to treat.

Hypothyroidism is more common in SLE than in the general population and should be considered in patients with severe lethargy.

Musculoskeletal features
Approximately 90% of patients with SLE experience arthralgia or arthritis, usually polyarticular. The

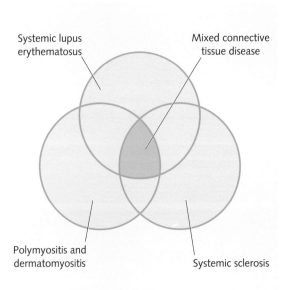

Fig. 11.1 Some members of the connective tissue disease family have overlapping features.

Factors capable of triggering flares of SLE
Overexposure to sunlight
Oestrogen-containing contraceptive therapy
Infection
Stress

Fig. 11.2 Factors capable of triggering flares of SLE.

arthritis is not erosive and the symptoms are usually more dramatic than the signs. If deformity occurs, it is due to tenosynovitis and fibrosis, rather than cartilage or bone erosion. Jaccoud's arthritis is the name given to this deformity in the hands, as it resembles the deformity of rheumatic fever.

Myalgia is a common symptom of SLE. Avascular necrosis of bone can occur, as can osteoporosis, but they are usually a consequence of corticosteroid treatment, rather than of the disease itself. Septic arthritis is a rare, serious, outcome.

Dermatological features

There are many cutaneous manifestations of lupus. Photosensitivity is common (c. 60%) The characteristic 'butterfly' rash develops over the nose and cheeks (Fig. 11.3). Discoid lupus (demarcated, pigmented or atrophic plaques) can develop with no systemic features (Fig. 11.4).

Hair loss reflects disease activity and alopecia may develop. Mucosal ulceration may affect the nose, mouth and vagina. Cutaneous vasculitis in SLE can present with urticarial lesions, livedo reticularis, palpable purpura and splinter haemorrhages.

Cardiovascular features

Serositis is common in SLE and pericarditis is the commonest cardiac manifestation. Myocarditis may accompany myositis and can present with arrhythmias or cardiac failure. Libman–Sacks endocarditis is due to non-infective vegetations and seldom causes clinical problems.

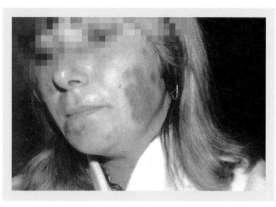

Fig. 11.4 Lesions of discoid lupus.

At least one-third of patients with SLE suffer from Raynaud's phenomenon. Vasospasm, usually provoked by the cold, causes peripheral ischaemia. This can be seen in the digits, tip of the nose and ear lobes, which become pale and numb, before turning blue. The final phase is of redness and flushing due to eventual vasodilatation. Vasculitis presents with skin rashes or ulcers and can rarely affect internal organs, such as the lungs and brain.

Pulmonary features

Amongst the pulmonary features of lupus, pleurisy and pleural effusions are common. Acute pneumonitis can mimic pneumonia. Chronic pneumonitis causes pulmonary fibrosis and presents with gradually increasing shortness of breath and a dry cough. Pulmonary hypertension is rare. When it does occur, emboli need to be excluded.

Renal features

Glomerulonephritis is the commonest cause of lupus-related death in patients with SLE. Nephritis does not cause clinical symptoms until there is significant renal damage. It is therefore important to monitor patients' blood pressure and check their urine for protein, red cells and casts, so that renal disease can be detected early.

Neurological features

SLE can involve the central nervous system, cranial and peripheral nerves, producing a wide range of clinical features. These include headaches, psychiatric problems, seizures, neuropathies and chorea. Headaches are common and often migrainous. Psychiatric symptoms such as anxiety, depression and psychosis are also well-recognized effects of lupus.

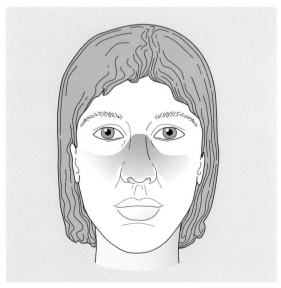

Fig. 11.3 The classic 'butterfly' rash of SLE.

Haematological features

Lymphopenia is usual in active SLE. It is sometimes difficult to distinguish whether other cytopenias, such as leucopenia and thrombocytopenia, are due to high disease activity or bone marrow suppression by drugs. Anaemia can be due to chronic inflammation or to autoimmune haemolysis, which affects at least 5% of lupus sufferers.

Gastrointestinal (GI) features

Aseptic peritonitis can present with abdominal pain and nausea, with or without ascites. Mild hepatosplenomegaly and vasculitis affecting the mesenteric vessels are other GI manifestations.

Overlap with other diseases

It is common for patients with SLE to develop secondary Sjögren's syndrome or the antiphospholipid antibody syndrome (see below).

Investigations
Serological tests

SLE is characterized by the presence of serum autoantibodies against nuclear components (see Fig. 11.5).

Other tests

- A full blood count should be performed regularly for anaemia, leucopenia and thrombocytopenia.
- The urine should be checked regularly with a dipstick to detect blood and protein. This is more sensitive than blood tests, although renal function should still be monitored by measuring serum urea, creatinine and electrolyte levels.
- The erythrocyte sedimentation rate (ESR) will rise during a flare of SLE (Fig. 11.6), but may sometimes be high when the patient feels quite well. The C-reactive protein (CRP) tends to

Indicators of high disease activity in SLE
Raised ESR High anti-DsDNA titres Low C3 and C4 complement levels

Fig. 11.6 Indicators of high disease activity in SLE.

remain normal unless infection, synovitis or serositis is present.

- Complement levels (C3 and C4) are usually depressed in active SLE.
- Coombs' test will be positive in patients with autoimmune haemolytic anaemia.
- Skin biopsy shows deposition of IgG and complement at the dermal–epidermal junction in patients with rashes (lupus 'band' test).
- Renal biopsy is sometimes performed to aid diagnosis or to establish prognosis in patients with abnormal renal function, when the relative contributions of active glomerular inflammation or irreversible damage can be assessed.

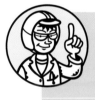

Always consider SLE as a possible diagnosis in a patient with multisystem symptoms, particularly if the patient has a raised ESR and normal CRP.

If the CRP rises in a patient with lupus, look for an infective source.

Fig. 11.5 Autoantibodies associated with SLE.

Autoantibodies associated with SLE	
Autoantibodies found in SLE	Comments
Antinuclear antibodies (ANA)	Detected in >95% of patients not specific for SLE
Anti-Ro and anti-La antibodies	Associated with secondary Sjögren's syndrome and pulmonary fibrosis Mothers are at risk of having babies with neonatal SLE and congenital heart block
Anti-double-stranded DNA (dsDNA) antibodies	Very specific for SLE A good marker of disease activity
Antihistone antibodies	Often positive in drug-induced SLE
Antiphospholipid and anticardiolipin antibodies	May be positive

Management
General measures
Education about SLE is essential. Patients are best advised to avoid factors that can precipitate lupus flares (see Fig. 11.2). They should wear long-sleeved clothes and use complete sunblock in any sunny weather. Infections should be promptly treated.

Pharmacological treatment
The choice of drug therapy in SLE depends on the severity and nature of the disease.

Mild SLE
Patients with symptoms such as arthralgia, lethargy or a faint rash may respond to non-steroidal anti-inflammatory drugs (NSAIDs) and/or antimalarial drugs, such as hydroxychloroquine. Long-term therapy with chloroquine carries a risk of retinal damage. Hydroxychloroquine has a very low risk of ocular toxicity, but it is probably still wise to arrange annual ophthalmological screening for patients taking the drug long term.

Moderate SLE
Patients with more severe clinical features, such as serositis, severe arthritis, nephritis, autoimmune haemolytic anaemia, thrombocytopenia and neurological or psychiatric problems often require treatment with corticosteroids. Steroid sparing with azathioprine or methotrexate is useful.

Severe SLE
Flares of SLE that cause severe renal, neurological or haematological problems should be treated with cytotoxic drugs combined with corticosteroids. Cyclophosphamide is the most effective but toxic. Others such as tacrolimus and mycophenolate mofetil may be alternatives.

Adjunctive treatment
Consider the individual requirements. Hypertension due to nephritis should be treated aggressively. Intravenous immunoglobulin infusions may help immune thrombocytopenia or neutropenia. Antiplatelet drugs or warfarin are required for those at risk. Osteoporosis should be anticipated. Anticonvulsants may be required in CNS disease.

Prognosis
The outlook for patients with SLE is improving. 5-year survival is at least 90%. When deaths do occur, they are usually a consequence of lupus nephritis,

although some are due to serious infections precipitated by cytotoxic drugs. However, with better control of inflammation, chronic organ damage is decreasing.

The antiphospholipid antibody syndrome

Definition
The antiphospholipid syndrome (APS) is characterized by recurrent vascular thrombosis, fetal loss and thrombocytopenia associated with persistently elevated levels of antiphospholipid antibodies (APA). APA production can complicate other autoimmune diseases, especially SLE. In these circumstances, patients are said to have secondary antiphospholipid antibody syndrome.

Incidence
APS was first described 20 years ago. It is increasingly being recognized as a cause of thrombosis, but its incidence and prevalence are still unclear.

Pathology
The two main antiphospholipid antibodies are lupus anticoagulant and anticardiolipin. Their role in thrombosis is currently being investigated. They appear to induce a procoagulant state by binding to antigens on endothelial cells. Placental infarction is thought to be the mechanism behind fetal loss.

Clinical features
The major features of antiphospholipid antibody syndrome are shown in Figure 11.7.

Patients with antiphospholipid antibody syndrome can develop additional clinical features to those shown above (see Fig. 11.8).

Investigations
The diagnosis is confirmed by finding lupus anticoagulant activity and/or anticardiolipin antibodies in the blood. Serological tests for syphilis (e.g. Venereal Disease Research Laboratory (VDRL)) are often false biological positives. Thrombocytopenia may occur.

The major features of APS	
Venous thrombosis	Deep vein thrombosis and pulmonary emboli—most common Other veins can be affected (e.g. inferior vena cava, pelvic, renal, portal and hepatic veins)
Arterial thrombosis	Cerebral ischaemia (stroke, transient ischaemic attacks) Peripheral ischaemia
Fetal complications	Spontaneous abortions—often in the 3rd trimester Premature births
Thrombocytopenia	Not severe enough to cause haemorrhage

Fig. 11.7 The major features of APS.

Associated clinical features of APS
Livedo reticularis Leg ulcers Cardiac valve abnormalities (e.g. aortic and mitral regurgitation) Chorea Epilepsy Migraine Haemolytic anaemia

Fig. 11.8 Associated clinical features of APS.

Management
General advice
The following steps are advisable:
- Avoidance of the oral contraceptive pill.
- Avoidance of smoking.
- Treatment of hypertension, hyperlipidaemia or diabetes.

Asymptomatic patients
Current recommendations are that patients with no history of thrombosis should be treated with low-dose aspirin.

Venous or arterial thrombosis
Patients with antiphospholipid antibody syndrome should be anticoagulated in the usual way. However, it is recommended that anticoagulation is lifelong, because there is a risk of recurrent thrombosis. Prophylactic therapy with warfarin, aiming for an international normalized ratio (INR) of 2.5–3.0 is recommended.

Recurrent fetal loss
Warfarin should be stopped before conception because it is teratogenic. Subcutaneous heparin should be given throughout pregnancy.

Sjögren's syndrome

Definition
Sjögren's syndrome is a chronic autoimmune disease, characterized by inflammation of exocrine glands. The salivary and lacrimal glands are predominantly affected, resulting in dryness of the eyes and mouth. Sjögren's syndrome can be primary or secondary (associated with other diseases). Causes of secondary Sjögren's syndrome are shown in Figure 11.9.

Prevalence
The prevalence of Sjögren's syndrome is 1–3%. It is nine times commoner in women.

Aetiology
The aetiology is unknown. The primary disease has a strong genetic association with HLA-DR3. It is thought that some environmental factor (probably a virus) may trigger Sjögren's syndrome in people with a genetic susceptibility.

Pathology
All organs affected by Sjögren's syndrome are infiltrated by lymphocytes. In the salivary glands, this results in duct dilatation, acinar atrophy and interstitial fibrosis. There is marked activation of

Diseases associated with secondary Sjögren's syndrome
RA SLE Systemic sclerosis Polymyositis Primary biliary cirrhosis Chronic active hepatitis

Fig. 11.9 Diseases associated with secondary Sjögren's syndrome.

B-cells, resulting in increased immunoglobulin production.

Clinical features

Sjögren's syndrome predominantly affects people in the fourth and fifth decades. The main symptoms are ocular or oral.

Ocular symptoms

Reduced tear secretion results in the destruction of the corneal and conjunctival epithelium (keratoconjunctivitis sicca). Patients complain that their eyes feel dry, sore or gritty and they are usually red. Bacterial conjunctivitis is common.

Oral symptoms

Xerostomia (dryness of the mouth) leads to difficulties in swallowing dry food or talking for long periods. Patients often take frequent sips of water to ease this. On examination of the oral cavity, the mucosa is dry, there is very little saliva and the tongue may be fissured. Dental caries is often seen and oral candidiasis is common. Intermittent parotid swelling affects at least half of patients with primary Sjögren's syndrome (Fig. 11.10), but is less common in secondary disease.

Other symptoms of exocrine dysfunction

Secretion from other exocrine glands may be diminished, producing a variety of clinical effects. For example, vaginal dryness can cause dyspareunia and lack of GI mucus secretion can result in oesophagitis or gastritis. There is an association with autoimmunity (e.g. thyroid disease).

Systemic features

Primary Sjögren's syndrome is a systemic disease and many patients develop extraglandular manifestations.

- Constitutional features include fatigue, weight loss and fever.
- Arthritis is episodic, non-erosive and very similar to the joint disease seen in SLE.
- Raynaud's phenomenon affects up to 50% of patients.
- Interstitial lung disease is mild and often subclinical.
- Interstitial nephritis can lead to renal tubular acidosis or nephrogenic diabetes insipidus.
- Vasculitis affects approximately 5% of patients and usually causes cutaneous lesions: purpura and ulcers.

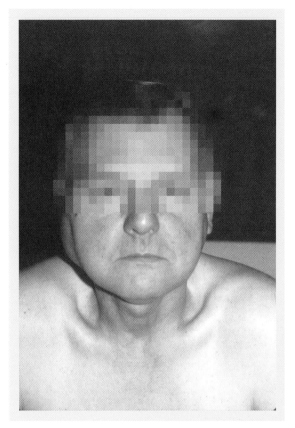

Fig. 11.10 Parotid swelling in Sjögren's syndrome.

- Neurological features vary widely. Peripheral neuropathies result from small vessel vasculitis. Cranial neuropathies, hemiparesis, seizures and movement disorders can also occur.
- Lymphomas, usually B-cell, are commoner in patients with Sjögren's syndrome than in the general population. They develop in the salivary glands, reticuloendothelial system, GI tract, lungs or kidneys.

Investigations
Schirmer's test

Schirmer's test is used to demonstrate reduced tear production. One end of a strip of filter paper is placed beneath the lower eyelid. The length of paper soaked by tears is measured after 5 minutes. Wetting of less than 5 mm suggests reduced secretion.

Rose Bengal staining

This is used to detect keratoconjunctivitis sicca. Rose Bengal is a dye that stains damaged corneal and conjunctival epithelium. This is seen clearly on slit-lamp examination.

Salivary flow rate monitoring
Salivary flow rate can be monitored with an isotope scan. This measures the rate at which a radiolabelled dye is taken up and excreted by the salivary glands. Both uptake and excretion are delayed in Sjögren's syndrome.

Labial gland biopsy and histology
Biopsy and histology of the labial glands from behind the lower lip is a very useful test. Lymphocytic infiltration can be seen.

Blood tests
- The ESR is usually high.
- A mild normocytic anaemia is common.
- Immunoglobulin levels are very high.
- Anti-Ro and anti-La antibodies, rheumatoid factor and antinuclear antibodies (ANA) are often found.

Do not assume that every patient with arthralgia and a positive rheumatoid factor has RA. Titres of rheumatoid factor can be very high in Sjögren's syndrome and patients with primary Sjögren's syndrome are often misdiagnosed as having RA.

Management
Treatment of Sjögren's syndrome is topical and symptomatic. Tear substitutes, such as hypromellose eye drops help to lubricate the eyes. Occlusion of the canaliculi can help to block the drainage of tears and keeps the conjunctiva moist.

Xerostomia can be treated with saliva substitutes. Pilocarpine tablets may help, but cause cholinergic side-effects such as sweating and abdominal cramps. Careful dental hygiene is essential to help prevent premature caries.

Hydroxychloroquine can help the arthritis. Corticosteroids are prescribed for serious complications like vasculitis and neurological problems. Cyclophosphamide can be added if patients do not respond.

Polymyositis and dermatomyositis

Definition
Polymyositis (PM) and dermatomyositis (DM) are autoimmune, inflammatory muscle diseases. DM also affects the skin.

Incidence
Both muscle diseases are rare, with a combined incidence of between 2–10 cases per million per year. There is a female preponderance of 2:1.

Aetiology
The aetiology of PM and DM is unknown. Family studies support a genetic predisposition. Associations with various HLA types have been reported, but are weak.

Pathology
In both conditions, muscle fibres are infiltrated by inflammatory cells and there is subsequent degeneration, necrosis and phagocytosis. The pattern of infiltration and predominant cell type allows PM to be distinguished from DM. Skin biopsy in DM shows the same histological features as in lupus. The autoantibodies commonly associated with inflammatory muscle disease will be discussed later.

Clinical features
Inflammatory muscle disease can affect people of any age, but the peak age of onset is 40–60 years. DM is often seen in children, but PM is unusual in this age group.

Myositis
PM and DM are characterized by symmetrical proximal muscle weakness that develops over weeks to months. Patients find certain tasks increasingly difficult, such as rising from a chair, climbing the stairs or reaching for things above head height.

Involvement of the intercostal muscles and diaphragm can affect ventilation and lead to type 2 respiratory failure. Dysphagia and regurgitation of food result from weakness of the pharyngeal muscles and upper third of the oesophagus. Patients may complain of muscle pain and tenderness. Muscle bulk and tendon reflexes appear normal, except in advanced disease.

Cutaneous manifestations
The skin rashes of DM usually precede the weakness. Typical lesions are:

- *Gottron's papules*—erythematous, scaly papules or plaques over the MCP and PIP joints and also over the extensor surfaces of the knees and elbows.
- A *heliotrope rash* develops on the skin over the eyelids; lilac discoloration is often accompanied by periorbital oedema.
- A *macular erythematous rash* may develop on the face, neck, chest, shoulders and hands.
- *Calcinosis*—this occurs more commonly in juvenile dermatomyositis than in adult disease.
- *Cutaneous vasculitis*—can cause ulceration
- *Periungual telangiectasia* may be seen and the cuticles are often thickened and irregular.

Some patients develop typical cutaneous features of DM without the muscle disease. They are said to have 'amyopathic DM'.

Extramuscular features of PM and DM
Constitutional features
Fatigue, malaise, weight loss and fever are common.

Skeletal features
Many patients develop polyarthralgia as well as myalgia.

Pulmonary features
Interstitial lung disease occurs in up to 30% of cases. Ventilatory failure can result from weakness of the intercostal muscles and diaphragm. Aspiration pneumonia is a risk in patients with dysphagia.

Cardiovascular features
Myocarditis can present with cardiac failure or arrhythmias, but most cases are asymptomatic. Raynaud's phenomenon and vasculitis can accompany myositis.

GI features
Vasculitis that can result in intestinal haemorrhage or perforation is particularly common in juvenile dermatomyositis.

Malignancy
Approximately 5–15% of adults with inflammatory muscle disease have an underlying malignancy. The association is thought to be much stronger for DM than for PM.

Malignancies reported in association with DM include:

- Lung.
- Oesophagus.
- Breast.
- Colon.
- Ovary.

Investigations
Serum levels of muscle enzymes
Serum levels of muscle enzymes are elevated due to myositis. The creatine kinase is measured most commonly and in active disease is at least 10 times the upper limit of normal.

Erythrocyte sedimentation rate
The ESR is usually raised, but does not correlate well with disease activity. Serum autoantibodies to nuclear and/or cytoplasmic antigens are found in more than 80% of patients. The ANA are usually positive. Approximately 30% of patients with PM or DM have myositis-specific antibodies. These can help predict a patient's prognosis and response to treatment. Anti-Jo-1 is an anticytoplasmic antibody and is associated with interstitial lung disease, arthralgia and Raynaud's phenomenon.

Muscle biopsy
This is the most definitive investigation. Histology shows the typical inflammatory cell infiltration of either PM or DM.

Electromyography and nerve conduction studies
Electromyography and nerve conduction studies can show that the weakness is due to a myopathic process, but do not give a specific diagnosis.

Magnetic resonance imaging
MRI can identify areas of muscle inflammation, but again is non-specific.

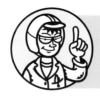
Adults with PM or DM should be screened for underlying malignancy.

Management
Corticosteroids are used to control myositis. They are initially prescribed at high doses. Serum creatine kinase is monitored and, once it is normal, the corticosteroid dose is gradually reduced. Although the muscle enzymes respond quickly to treatment, the improvement in muscle strength is usually much slower. Many patients with PM or DM require

additional immunosuppressive therapy. Methotrexate and azathioprine are commonly used. Cyclophosphamide may be prescribed for patients with severe interstitial lung disease.

Physiotherapy plays an extremely important role in the rehabilitation of patients with inflammatory muscle disease. If an underlying malignancy is found, it should be treated appropriately.

Steroid myopathy is a common complication of treatment. It may be difficult to distinguish from active myositis, but should be considered in patients with normal creatine kinase levels whose muscle strength is deteriorating.

Prognosis

The 5-year survival rate of patients with PM and DM has improved and is currently over 80%. However, many patients are left with significant persisting symptoms as a result of their disease or therapy.

Systemic sclerosis and related conditions

Definition

The term 'scleroderma' means hardening of the skin. This is a feature of several disorders (see Fig. 11.11). Localized cutaneous scleroderma is confined to the skin and soft tissues, whereas systemic sclerosis (SSc) involves internal organs as well.

Incidence and prevalence

These are rare conditions. The incidence of scleroderma is 0.6–1.9 per million per year. The UK prevalence is approximately 100 per million. Women are affected four times as often as men.

Aetiology

In most patients, the aetiology is unknown. Specific HLA types are associated with certain subsets of disease, but not with the disease as a whole. Exposure to certain chemicals or drugs has been associated with SSc.

Classification of systemic sclerosis and related conditions
Localized cutaneous scleroderma Morphoea Linear scleroderma
Systemic sclerosis Limited cutaneous systemic sclerosis Diffuse cutaneous systemic sclerosis Scleroderma *sine* scleroderma

Fig. 11.11 Classification of systemic sclerosis and related conditions.

Pathology

The two main pathological processes in SSc are fibrosis and microvascular occlusion. Overactive fibroblasts produce excessive extracellular matrix in the dermis. Perivascular inflammatory infiltration and intimal proliferation lead to narrowing of arteries and arterioles and obliteration of capillaries. There is immune activation and release of cytokines.

Clinical features
Localized cutaneous scleroderma

Localized scleroderma presents with painful, erythematous lesions, which later become fibrotic. The two main types are morphoea and linear scleroderma. Morphoea varies from small, discrete lesions to large, confluent patches that are uncomfortable and disfiguring. Linear scleroderma is commoner in childhood. Bands of sclerosis affect the limbs and lead to growth defects.

Systemic sclerosis

In addition to causing disfiguring skin changes, SSc can have profound effects on many other organs. The disease is divided into limited cutaneous SSc and diffuse cutaneous SSc. Limited disease is twice as common as diffuse and is sometimes referred to as CREST syndrome (CREST = Calcinosis, Raynaud's, oEsophageal disease, Sclerodactyly and Telangiectasia).

Symptoms develop most commonly in the fifth decade of life.

Skin manifestations

Scleroderma begins with an inflammatory phase. The skin becomes puffy and feels tight and sometimes itchy. These symptoms typically affect the forearms, hands and feet initially. Over several months, skin thickening and induration develop.

Common features found on examination are:
- Sclerodactyly (Fig. 11.12).
- Microstomia (Fig. 11.13).
- Furrowing of skin around the lips (Fig. 11.13).

- Loss of normal skin creases.
- Tethering of skin to underlying structures.
- Skin hypo- or hyperpigmentation.
- Flexion contractures of joints.

In the late stages of scleroderma, the skin becomes thin and atrophic.

The skin changes differ between diffuse and limited cutaneous systemic sclerosis. The main differences are outlined in Figure 11.14.

The effects of systemic sclerosis on other body systems

Involvement of internal organs is more frequent in diffuse than in limited disease.

Cardiovascular manifestations

Raynaud's phenomenon This occurs in nearly every case of SSc. Severe disease may cause ischaemic changes in the fingertips and possibly gangrene. The toes, ears, nose and nipples can also be involved.

Cardiac disease Disease is due to myocardial or pericardial involvement. Myocardial fibrosis can cause cardiac failure and arrhythmias. Pericarditis is often clinically silent.

Pulmonary disease

Pulmonary disease is the most frequent cause of death in SSc. It can take the form of interstitial fibrosis or pulmonary vascular disease.

Fibrosing alveolitis This affects approximately 25% of patients with limited disease and up to 40% of those with the diffuse cutaneous form.

Pulmonary hypertension This affects 10–20% of patients. It can be primary (not associated with other lung pathology) or secondary to pulmonary fibrosis.

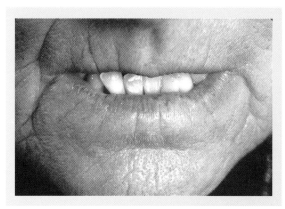

Fig. 11.12 This patient with systemic sclerosis has microstomia and furrowing of the skin around her mouth.

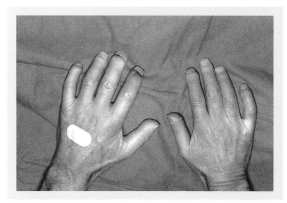

Fig. 11.13 Sclerodactyly.

Primary pulmonary hypertension is more common in limited cutaneous SSc, and secondary pulmonary hypertension is more common in diffuse cutaneous SSc.

Fig. 11.14 A comparison of skin disease between limited and diffuse systemic sclerosis.

A comparison of skin disease between limited and diffuse cutaneous systemic sclerosis		
	Limited systemic sclerosis	Diffuse systemic sclerosis
Distribution of skin fibrosis	Hands* and feet Over the face and neck	Limbs, face, neck and trunk
Skin tethering to underlying structures	Common	Less common
Inflammatory features	Mild	Swelling and pruritus prominent
Telangiectasia	Commonly occur on the face and digits	Less common
Calcinosis	Cutaneous and subcutaneous Calcification common	Less common

Scleroderma affecting the fingers is often referred to as 'sclerodactyly'

Renal disease

Scleroderma renal crisis This implies rapidly progressive renal failure, usually with accelerated hypertension. It tends to occur in patients with diffuse cutaneous disease within 5 years of onset and is often preceded by deterioration of skin disease. Patients present acutely with headaches, visual disturbance and, sometimes, fits due to accelerated hypertension. Left ventricular failure can occur and death from renal failure is likely without rapid intervention.

 Scleroderma renal crisis is a life-threatening medical emergency that needs urgent treatment.

GI manifestations

Scleroderma can affect any part of the GI tract, but oesophageal problems are particularly common. Reflux oesophagitis and oesophageal dysmotility cause heartburn and dysphagia. Hypomotility can cause bacterial overgrowth in the small bowel and constipation in the large bowel.

Musculoskeletal complications

Most patients suffer with arthralgia and joint stiffness at some time in their disease. Flexion contractures of the interphalangeal joints are common.

Scleroderma *sine* scleroderma

A small minority of patients have the typical vascular or internal organ features of systemic sclerosis without skin sclerosis. They are said to have scleroderma *sine* scleroderma.

Investigations

The diagnosis of scleroderma is clinical. It is important to establish whether patients with SSc have diffuse or limited disease, as this determines prognosis.

Serological tests

Antinuclear antibodies are found in 95% of patients. The presence or absence of other autoantibodies can help predict complications and prognosis.

For example:

- Anticentromere antibodies are associated with limited disease and a relatively good prognosis. They signify a risk of pulmonary hypertension, but not pulmonary fibrosis.

- Antitopoisomerase-1 (Scl-70) antibodies are associated with diffuse disease and a higher risk of lung fibrosis and renal involvement.

Management

Disease-modifying and antifibrotic therapy

Researchers are still trying to find effective therapies to modify the disease process underlying SSc. Many drugs that affect the immune response have been tested, but none has been very effective. Antifibrotic drugs, such as penicillamine and interferon-α may help prevent visceral and skin fibrosis if given early.

Screening for complications

This is a very important part in the management of SSc. The blood pressure and renal function should be regularly monitored. Pulmonary function tests and echocardiography will help to detect pulmonary involvement.

Treatment of complications

A lot can be done to treat the organ-related complications. Please see Figure 11.15.

Prognosis

The survival of patients with systemic sclerosis is improving. This probably reflects better management of complications. Estimates of the 5-year survival rate range from 35–70% in studies.

The vasculitides

Definition

Vasculitis is inflammation of blood vessels. It is a feature of many illnesses and can be primary or secondary. The primary vasculitides are uncommon diseases in which vasculitis is the predominant feature. Secondary vasculitis complicates other established diseases such as rheumatoid arthritis (RA), systemic lupus erythematosus (SLE) or HIV infection. Only primary vasculitis will be discussed here.

Aetiopathology

Vasculitis is characterized by inflammatory cell infiltration of the blood vessel wall, resulting in fibrinoid necrosis. For this reason, the term 'necrotizing vasculitis' is sometimes used. There is often associated granuloma formation. Vascular inflammation can have severe consequences:

- Aneurysm formation can lead to rupture of vessels and haemorrhage.

Fig. 11.15 Treatment of internal organ disease in systemic sclerosis.

Treatment of internal organ disease in systemic sclerosis	
Complication	**Intervention**
Raynaud's phenomenon	Handwarmers Vasodilators • Calcium-channel blockers • ACE inhibitors • Intravenous prostacyclin (iloprost) for severe ischaemia Digital sympathectomy is useful for ischaemia of one or two Digits
Pulmonary fibrosis	Prednisolone, with or without cyclophosphamide
Pulmonary hypertension	Anticoagulation Vasodilators • Calcium-channel blockers • Prostacyclin Diuretics for right ventricular failure, if present
Gastrointestinal problems	Proton pump inhibitor for gastro-oesophageal reflux Antibiotics for small bowel overgrowth Bulk-forming agents for constipation
Renal crisis	Antihypertensives—give immediately • ACE inhibitors • Calcium-channel blockers Temporary dialysis may be required
Cardiac problems	Diuretics and ACE inhibitors for cardiac failure Antiarrhythmics if necessary Corticosteroids for myocarditis

• Vessel stenosis or occlusion can lead to distal infarction.

Antineutrophil cytoplasmic antibodies (ANCA) are particularly specific for vasculitis and are helpful for diagnosis and classification. They are antibodies that bind to antigens in the cytoplasm of neutrophils. There are two types of ANCA:

• Cytoplasmic ANCA (c-ANCA) is found in patients with Wegener's granulomatosis and is highly specific.
• Perinuclear staining ANCA (p-ANCA) is found in polyarteritis nodosa, microscopic polyangiitis and Churg–Strauss syndrome.

Classification of primary vasculitis

The vasculitides are commonly classified on the basis of the size of the vessels they affect (Fig. 11.16).

Clinical features

It is important to have a good understanding of the clinical effects of vasculitis and to know when to suspect it. Many types of primary vasculitis are rare, and detailed knowledge of these individual diseases is beyond the scope of this book. This section will therefore discuss the effects of vasculitis in general, then describe the diseases, allocating the most space to those that occur more frequently.

Classification of primary vasculitis

Large vessel vasculitis
Giant cell (temporal) arteritis and polymyalgia rheumatica
Takayasu's arteritis

Medium vessel vasculitis
Polyarteritis nodosa
Kawasaki's disease

Small vessel vasculitis
Wegener's granulomatosis*
Churg–Strauss syndrome*
Microscopic polyangiitis*
Henoch–Schönlein purpura
Essential cryoglobulinaemic vasculitis

Vasculitides most commonly associated with ANCA

Fig. 11.16 Classification of primary vasculitis.

Vasculitis is potentially life-threatening. The clinical features depend on the size, site and number of blood vessels involved. The most serious problems are due to haemorrhage or infarction of internal organs.

Constitutional features

All primary vasculitic illnesses can cause systemic upset. Features such as fatigue, anorexia, weight loss and fever are common.

Features due to involvement of different body systems

Vasculitis can affect any system of the body (Fig. 11.17).

Giant cell arteritis (GCA) and polymyalgia rheumatica (PMR)
Clinical features

These related diseases are the commonest types of primary vasculitis, with an incidence of approximately 1–5 in 10 000. They both target people over 60 years of age and are twice as common in females than in males. About 50% of patients with GCA have symptoms of PMR and 20–50% of patients with PMR have GCA symptoms.

GCA

Most symptoms are due to inflammation of the carotid artery or its branches, although other large arteries can be involved. The onset of GCA is fairly abrupt, with symptoms often appearing overnight. Patients complain of headache, scalp tenderness and sometimes pain on chewing food (jaw claudication). The temporal artery is thickened and tender on examination, sometimes with absent pulsation.

The most feared complication of GCA is blindness. This is due to ischaemic optic neuritis, caused by arteritis of the posterior ciliary and branches of the ophthalmic arteries. Patients may experience transient disturbance of vision first. Stroke is another serious potential complication.

PMR

Patients present with symmetrical pain and stiffness in the shoulder and pelvic girdles. Proximal muscles are weak and may be tender. Peripheral synovitis affecting medium-sized joints is common.

Investigations

The diagnosis of PMR is clinical. It is important to exclude malignancy and other connective tissue diseases, which can mimic PMR.

Temporal artery biopsy is the investigation of choice for GCA, but it is not always helpful. The arteritis is patchy and if a 'skip lesion' is biopsied, histology will be normal. Inflammatory cell infiltration, giant cells and granulomata should be seen.

The ESR is usually raised in both conditions, often to at least 70 mm/h. However, a normal ESR does not exclude the diagnoses. Anaemia is common.

The effects that vasculitis can have on different body systems	
Body system or organ	**Manifestations of vasculitis**
Skin	Rashes Palpable purpura Ulceration Ischaemia [Fig. 11.18]
Joints	Arthralgia Arthritis
Kidneys	Glomerulonephritis
GI tract	Ischaemia
Nervous system	Neuropathies Stroke
Lungs	Pulmonary haemorrhage

Fig. 11.17 The effects that vasculitis can have on different body systems.

 Steroids reduce the inflammatory infiltrate within days, so if possible the biopsy should be done before treatment.

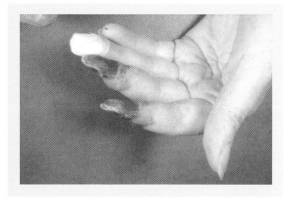

Fig. 11.18 Ischaemic changes in the fingers of a patient with vasculitis.

Management

Both GCA and PMR should be treated with corticosteroids. Prednisolone at a dose of 10–20 mg is usually prescribed for PMR. Higher doses are required for GCA, particularly in patients with visual symptoms.

There is usually a dramatic response to steroid therapy with symptoms improving after the first few doses. Once the disease activity has been completely suppressed, the corticosteroid dose can be gradually

Corticosteroid dose reduction should be guided by clinical features, not ESR.

tapered. The slower the dose reduction is, the less likely the patient is to relapse. Azathioprine and methotrexate are sometimes used as steroid-sparing agents if weaning off prednisolone is proving difficult.

Most patients with GCA or PMR will be taking corticosteroids for at least 1 year. Prescription of bone-protective drugs for the prevention of osteoporosis should be considered.

Takayasu's arteritis

This is a rare disease that predominantly affects young women. The arteritis affects the aortic arch and its branches. Symptoms are due to vascular ischaemia and include claudication, dizziness, visual loss and stroke. Immunosuppression may help the acute symptoms. Vascular surgery is often required to bypass obliterated vessels.

Polyarteritis nodosa

Polyarteritis nodosa is a necrotizing arteritis that leads to aneurysm formation. It affects men more frequently than it does women. Some cases are associated with hepatitis B infection. Clinical features include skin ulceration and rashes, peripheral neuropathy, renal disease and gut infarction, which presents with bleeding and abdominal pain. Angiography may show microaneurysms, which are usually found in renal arteries and the coeliac axis. Renal, rectal or sural nerve biopsies can be diagnostic.

Polyarteritis nodosa is treated with steroids and immunosuppressants. Cyclophosphamide is usually used and has improved prognosis.

Kawasaki's disease (mucocutaneous lymph node syndrome)

This vasculitis predominantly affects children under the age of 5 years. It was first described in Japan, where most cases occur. It is rare in the western world. Systemic symptoms are prominent. Other features include desquamation of the skin of the hands and feet, conjunctival congestion, cervical lymphadenopathy, arthritis and coronary arteritis, which can lead to acute myocardial infarction.

Wegener's granulomatosis

Wegener's granulomatosis is a granulomatous disorder associated with necrotizing vasculitis. It is strongly linked with the presence of c-ANCA. The peak age of onset is in the fourth and fifth decades. Many systems can be affected (Fig. 11.19), but it is

Fig. 11.19 Clinical features of Wegener's granulomatosis.

Clinical features of Wegener's granulomatosis	
Body system or organ affected	Clinical features
Upper and lower respiratory tracts	Stridor Lung nodules ± cavitation Pulmonary haemorrhage
Kidneys	Glomerulonephritis (often rapidly progressive)
Ear, nose and throat	Sensorineural deafness Nasal discharge, crusting and epistaxis 'Saddling' of the nose due to destruction of the Septal cartilage (Fig. 11.20)
Joints	Arthralgia Arthritis
Skin	Rashes Palpable purpura Livedo reticularis
Nervous system	Cranial nerve palsies Peripheral neuropathy Granulomatous meningitis

respiratory and renal complications that are the most serious. Many clinical features of granuloma formation are due to destruction or compression of surrounding structures.

Survival in Wegener's granulomatosis has improved dramatically since the introduction of cyclophosphamide therapy, which is given in conjunction with corticosteroids for most cases. Some patients with limited, non-life-threatening Wegener's granulomatosis can be treated less aggressively.

Churg–Strauss syndrome

In Churg–Strauss syndrome, granulomatous, necrotizing vasculitis is found in association with asthma and eosinophilia. Recurrent pneumonia, heart failure, skin lesions, mild renal impairment and peripheral neuropathies can also occur.

Microscopic polyangiitis

Severe renal disease is the main feature of microscopic polyangiitis. Rashes, arthralgia and myalgia are common and lung involvement can present with asthma, pleurisy or haemoptysis.

Henoch–Schönlein purpura

This vasculitis predominantly affects children. It typically involves the skin, gut, kidneys and joints. Patients can present with a purpuric rash, arthritis, gastrointestinal haemorrhage, abdominal pain and glomerulonephritis.

Essential cryoglobulinaemic vasculitis

This rare vasculitis presents with purpuric skin lesions, arthralgia and renal disease.

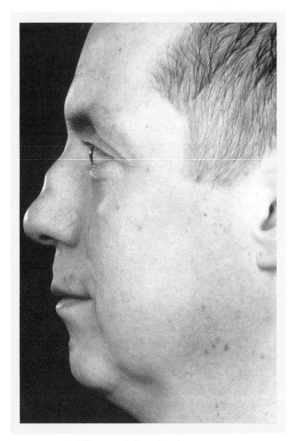

Fig. 11.20 Saddle nose deformity of Wegener's granulomatosis.

- Name three drugs that can cause drug-induced systemic lupus erythematosus (SLE).
- Which autoantibodies are commonly found in the serum of patients with SLE?
- Which blood tests can indicate increased disease activity in SLE?
- Discuss the three major features of the antiphospholipid antibody syndrome.
- What diseases are associated with secondary Sjögren's syndrome?
- What tests are used in the diagnosis of Sjögren's syndrome?
- What are the dermatological manifestations of dermatomyositis?
- Describe the differences between diffuse and limited cutaneous systemic sclerosis.
- What are the life-threatening complications of systemic sclerosis?
- What are the symptoms of giant cell arteritis?
- How are giant cell arteritis and polymyalgia rheumatica treated?

Further reading

Ball E and Louis Bridges S Jr 2002 *Vasculitis*. Oxford University Press, Oxford

Callen J P 2000 Dermatomyositis. *Lancet* **355**: 53-57

Denton C P, Black C M 2000 Scleroderma and related disorders: therapeutic aspects. *Bailliere's Best Pract Res Clin Rheumatol.* **14**(1): 17-35

Hazleman B L 2003 Polymyalgia rheumatica and giant cell arteritis. In: Hochberg et al (eds) *Rheumatology*, 3rd edn. Mosby, London, p 1623-1634

Hughes G 1999 *Lupus, the facts*. Oxford University Press, Oxford

Maddison P Is it a Connective Tissue Disease? In: *ABC of Rheumatology*, 3rd edn. BMJ Books, London

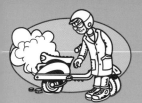

12. Osteoporosis and Metabolic Bone Disease

Osteoporosis

Because of the ageing population, fractures resulting from osteoporosis put enormous pressure on hospital services and incur vast costs. In the UK the number of hip fractures is increasing at 6% per year.

Definition
Osteoporosis is a skeletal disorder characterized by decreased bone strength leading to increased risk of fracture.

Osteopenia is a term used to describe low bone density but not severe enough to be called osteoporosis.

Incidence
Osteoporosis is very common and is predominantly a disease of elderly females.

45% of women over the age of 80 will have evidence of a vertebral fracture indicating osteoporosis.

Aetiology and pathology
There are certain aetiological factors in the development of osteoporosis over which the individual has no control, such as female sex, family history, early menopause, small size and Caucasian race. However, there are other factors such as level of exercise during adolescence and early adulthood (building good bone stock), smoking, alcohol intake, and weight-bearing exercise over which the individual can have some influence.

The development of osteoporosis is related to the amount of 'bone stock' the individual retains. Figure 12.1 gives a bone lifeline.

We divide osteoporosis into:
- Primary (age related and postmenopausal), or.
- Secondary (resulting from another disease process).

In both, the pathology is related to the balance between the osteoblast (cell producing bone) and the osteoclast (cell removing bone).

An imbalance results between these cell lines, producing a net loss of bone. Primary osteoporosis relates to the effects of cell ageing with less bone

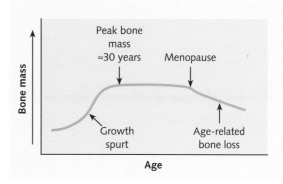

Fig. 12.1 'Lifeline' of bone mass.

produced in elderly patients and also to the effect of the menopause on oestrogen production.

Oestrogen has a positive effect on osteoblasts and therefore as oestrogen levels drop so does bone production (Fig. 12.2).

Other causes of secondary osteoporosis include rheumatoid arthritis, endocrine disorders (hyperparathyroidism, hypercortisolism, hyperthyroidism, testosterone deficiency), myeloma, drugs, e.g. corticosteroids, and immobility.

Cancellous bone is affected more than cortical bone and histologically we see thinning of trabeculae, decreased size of osteons and enlargement of haversian canals.

Clinical features
Osteoporosis is usually asymptomatic until fracture occurs.
- Patients can present with a deformity such as a kyphosis of the spine secondary to vertebral wedge compression fractures.
- The patient may also notice loss of height.
- Pain is usually only present in impending or actual fracture.
- Any patient presenting with a fracture after low-trauma injury should be suspected of having osteoporosis. Younger patients are more likely to have secondary osteoporosis.

Diagnosis and investigation
- In most cases the first investigation performed will be an X-ray because the patient has a fracture.

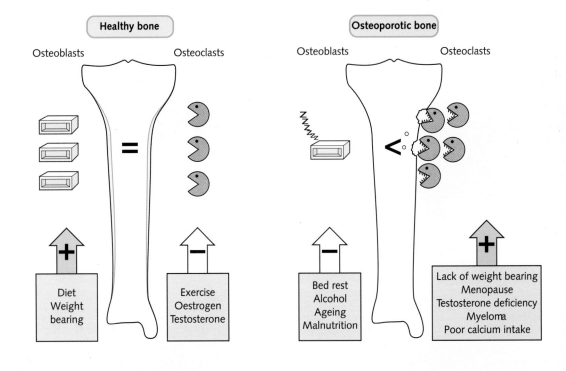

Fig. 12.2 Cell interactions in normal and osteoporotic bone.

X-rays can give an indication of osteopenia, particularly if it is severe, but cannot accurately diagnose osteoporosis.

- A DEXA scan (dual energy X-ray absorptiometry) by measuring bone mineral density is the most accurate way to diagnose osteoporosis and indicates the severity, therefore giving a fracture risk.
- Heel ultrasound bone densitometry is also used in some centres.
- In all cases serum calcium should be checked, as hyperparathyroidism can present with osteoporosis. Other investigations may target endocrine causes suspected in certain patients.

Management

The aim is to prevent fracture by preserving bone stock. Prevention is better than cure as the majority of patients present too late, having already fractured!

General advice should be given about maintaining a diet that is rich in vitamin D, calcium and protein. Regular weight-bearing exercise should be continued throughout life.

Stopping smoking and reducing alcohol intake also helps.

Treatment depends on the age of the patient, severity of osteoporosis and other risk factors (Fig. 12.3). Protocols are now followed to guide treatment.

Starting perimenopausal women on hormone-replacement therapy early (within 6 years) to preserve bone has obvious benefits but there are cardiovascular risks and links with breast cancer.

In the elderly population (particularly the immobile) vitamin D and calcium supplements should be routinely prescribed if an osteoporotic fracture occurs.

In more mobile patients with proven osteoporosis on DEXA scan bisphosphonates such as risedronate are now routinely prescribed. These drugs act by inhibiting osteoclastic activity.

Other agents such as raloxifene (a selective oestrogen receptor modulator), calcitonin and parathyroid hormone may have a role in certain cases.

Risk factors for fracture
Previous fracture (most important)
Low body weight
Immobility
Age >75
Female sex
Associated disorders
Malnutrition
Corticosteroid therapy
Alcoholism

Fig. 12.3 Risk factors for fracture.

Osteoporotic fractures

The three most common osteoporotic fractures are of the spine, wrist and hip.

All result from low-energy injuries in an elderly population. Some consideration must be given as to why elderly patients fall.

Falls in the elderly may occur for the following reasons:
1. Intrinsic factors:
   - Ageing process—leads to slower reaction times (patients unable to stop falling)
   - Poor mobility—patients often have other conditions such as OA
   - Poor eyesight
   - Medical co-morbidity, e.g. syncope/cardiac arrhythmia.
2. Extrinsic factors:
   - Lack of social services
   - Inadequate housing/unsafe local environment.

Unexplained falls in the elderly must be investigated!

Spine

Osteoporotic fractures of the spine are vertebral wedge compression fractures (Fig. 12.4). Usually they present as thoracic back pain after a minor fall. Often they are asymptomatic, frequently multiple and result in loss of height and a kyphotic deformity.

These are stable fractures and treatment is therefore aimed at controlling symptoms with analgesia and mobilizing the patient. Braces are sometimes used but are poorly tolerated.

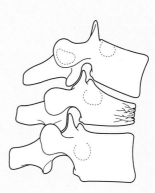

Fig. 12.4 Compression fracture of a thoracic vertebra (from Dandy, 1998).

The underlying osteoporosis needs treatment as spine fractures are a warning sign of future hip fracture.

New treatments include balloon vertebroplasty, where a catheter is inserted into the vertebral body and cement is injected into the space, preventing a fracture.

Wrist

The Colles' fracture is more common and results from a fall onto the outstretched hand (FOOSH) resulting in a dinner fork deformity. There is dorsal angulation and displacement of the fracture with also radial angulation and shortening (Fig. 12.5).

When managing a patient with a Colles' fracture it is important to assess the patient's general condition before concentrating on the fractured limb.

Condition of the skin and distal neurovascular status are noted.

The fracture is usually manipulated under local or regional anaesthetic and placed into a plaster cast.

More complex fractures may require surgery as outlined in Chapter 15, particularly in well, active patients.

The Smith's fracture is displaced in the opposite direction, i.e. volar or palmar displacement (Fig. 12.5). Such fractures are usually the result of a fall onto a flexed wrist.

Treatment of a Smith's fracture is difficult in a plaster cast alone and the position is often lost leading to a malunion and poor function.

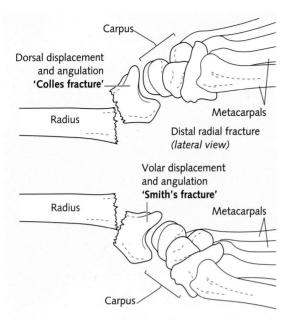

Fig. 12.5 Common osteoporotic distal radial fractures (lateral view).

Most centres would now treat a Smith's fracture with internal fixation.

Hip

Of the three common types of osteoporotic fracture, hip fractures place the greatest demand on resources and have the greatest impact on patients in terms of mortality, disability and loss of independence (approximately one-third of patients with a hip fracture will die within 1 year of injury).

Hip protectors can reduce the risk of fracture in nursing home patients but in practice they are too bulky and are rarely used because of lack of compliance.

In the vast majority of cases, femoral neck fractures are treated surgically rather than conservatively. The risk of surgery is balanced against the risks of prolonged bed rest or traction, such as bedsores, deep vein thrombosis and pneumonia.

Postoperative patients are mobilized early to minimize these complications. Even when faced with a bed-bound nursing home resident we still usually operate to provide pain relief and for ease of nursing/hygiene.

Hip fractures can be divided into:
- Intracapsular fractures.
- Extracapsular fractures.

The most important distinguishing feature is the blood supply to the femoral head. The blood supply enters the head through the capsule, therefore:

- In an intracapsular fracture (Fig. 12.6A and B), the fracture line is between the blood supply and the head, leading to a risk of avascular necrosis.
- In an extracapsular fracture (Fig. 12.6C), the head is in continuity with its blood supply and therefore the head does not have a risk of avascular necrosis.

This pathophysiology guides the treatment.

Intracapsular fractures can be divided into undisplaced and displaced.
- Undisplaced fractures can be treated with internal fixation.
- Displaced fractures (Figs 12.6 and 12.7) are treated with hemiarthroplasty, the femoral head being removed, leaving the artificial head articulating with the normal acetabulum.

Extracapsular fractures are trochanteric (Fig. 12.8) or subtrochanteric and are treated with internal fixation with either a dynamic hip screw or an intramedullary nail.

 The subtrochanteric region is a common place for metastatic deposits and care must be taken not to miss these.

Paget's disease

Definition

Paget's disease is a localized grossly deforming bone-remodelling disorder.

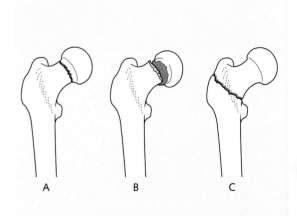

Fig. 12.6 Fractures of the femoral neck: (A) undisplaced intracapsular fracture; (B) displaced intracapsular fracture; (C) extracapsular trochanteric fracture.

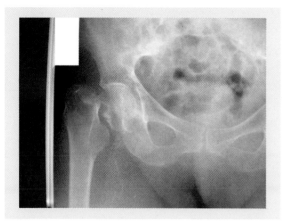

Fig. 12.7 Displaced intracapsular hip fracture.

Incidence

3% of the population > 40 years are affected by the disease. Of these, the majority will be asymptomatic and only 1 in 20 will complain of pain.

Aetiology

Geographically Paget's is most commonly found in western Europe and the US and there is clearly a genetic component involved. We do not know the exact cause yet but a viral infection is strongly implicated.

Pathology

Abnormally large multinucleated osteoclasts are markedly increased in number and activity causing bone resorption (Fig. 12.9). Osteoblasts then respond in turn, producing weak disorganized woven bone. This sequence of events is repeated several times producing abnormally large deformed bones with increased vascularity.

Clinical features

Patients with Paget's disease present in one of three ways:

1. symptomatic patients complain of pain, warmth and tenderness over the affected limb; the sites commonly involved are summarized in Figure 12.10
2. with a complication such as fracture or deformity
3. as an incidental finding.

Diagnosis and investigation

- Biochemistry shows a greatly elevated alkaline phosphatase level.
- Radiographic findings include disorganized pattern of bone with areas of lysis and sclerosis. The cortex is thickened and the medullary cavity narrowed.

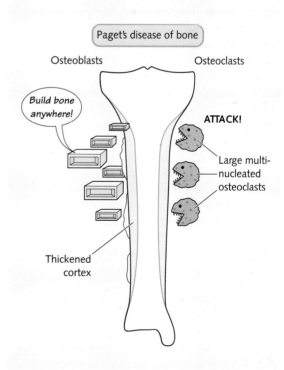

Fig. 12.9 Cell interactions in Paget's disease of bone.

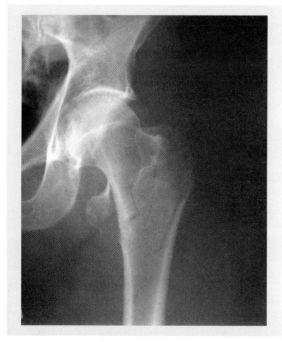

Fig. 12.8 Trochanteric hip fracture.

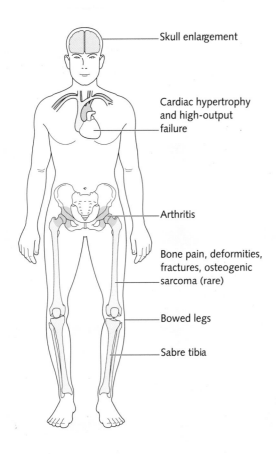

- Skull enlargement

- Cardiac hypertrophy and high-output failure

- Arthritis

- Bone pain, deformities, fractures, osteogenic sarcoma (rare)

- Bowed legs

- Sabre tibia

Fig. 12.10 Sites commonly involved in Paget's disease of bone.

Treatment

Medical treatment with bisphosphonates, such as risedronate, is very effective at reducing bone turnover and relieving patients' symptoms.

Surgical treatment is reserved for complications of:
- Fracture—needs surgical stabilization.
- Deformity—osteotomy rarely performed.
- Osteosarcoma—these tumours are highly aggressive with a poor prognosis. If the appendicular skeleton is involved, resection or amputation with chemotherapy is required.

 Pagetic bone is very vascular and bleeds a lot during surgery. Make sure the patient has blood available.

Osteomalacia and rickets

Both of these conditions are the result of failure of mineralization of bone resulting from vitamin D deficiency, leaving weak osteoid. Rickets occurs in children and osteomalacia in adults.

Aetiology

The conditions are rare in Caucasians but are seen particularly in Asian immigrants and also in the developing world.

They are due to:
1. nutritional deficiency: vitamin D, chelators or antacid abuse
2. gastrointestinal (GI) absorption defects, e.g. post-gastrectomy or biliary disease
3. renal disease.

Lack of sunlight is an additional factor.

Pathology

The active metabolite of vitamin D aids absorption of calcium from the GI tract and also influences osteoclastic activity on bone (Fig. 12.11).

In the absence of vitamin D the body responds by producing excess parathyroid hormone to raise levels of calcium in the blood. This so-called secondary hyperparathyroidism explains some of the features of rickets and osteomalacia.

Important histological findings in rickets and osteomalacia include 'Swiss cheese' trabeculae and widened osteoid seams.

Additionally, rickets as a disease of childhood affects the growth plate with distortion of the physis and poorly defined calcification.

The long bones show thickening and widening of physes, cupping and widening of the metaphysis and bowing of the diaphysis.

In osteomalacia the pathognomonic feature is stress fractures through weight-bearing bone called 'Looser's zones'.

Clinical features

Adults and children may complain of aches and pains and also generalized weakness.

Children with rickets have thickening of wrists, bow legs, stunted growth, coxa vara and occasionally tetany and convulsions.

Adults get stress fractures.

Diagnosis and investigation

- Blood tests will show decreased calcium and phosphate and increased alkaline phosphatase.
- X-rays show the features explained above.

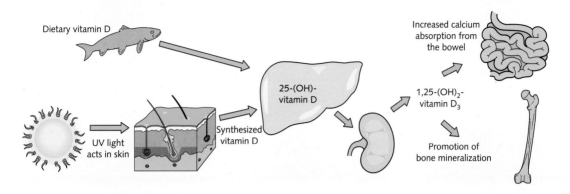

Fig. 12.11 Formation and actions of vitamin D.

Treatment
The condition almost always responds well to vitamin D supplementation.

Providing the child is young enough, even significant deformities should 'grow out' over time and corrective osteotomy is rarely indicated.

- What is osteoporosis?
- What are the risk factors for osteoporotic fractures?
- Describe the three most common osteoporotic fractures?
- How do you treat osteoporosis?
- Why do the elderly have so many fractures?
- What is Paget's disease?
- What are the complications of Paget's disease?
- Outline the role osteoclasts and osteoblasts play in Paget's disease and osteoporosis?
- Describe osteomalacia and rickets?
- How do you treat rickets and osteomalacia?

Further reading
Dandy D J 1998 Essentials of orthopaedics and trauma, 3rd edn. Churchill Livingstone, London
Fitzgerald R H, Kaufer H, Malkani A (eds) 2002 Orthopaedics. Mosby, Philadelphia
Miller M D 2000 Review of orthopaedics, 3rd edn. WB Saunders, Philadelphia

Solomon L, Warwick D, Nayagan D (eds) 2001 Apley's system of orthopaedics and fractures, 8th edn. Hodder Arnold, London
Orthoteers website: http://www.orthoteers.co.uk

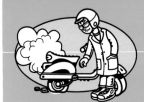

13. Crystal Arthropathies

Gout

Definition
Gout is a consequence of hyperuricaemia and uric acid crystal formation. Clinical features include:
- Arthritis.
- Crystal deposition in the soft tissues.
- Renal disease.
- Urolithiasis.

Prevalence
Gout affects between 0.5 and 2.5% of people in the western world. It used to be at least 10 times more common in men than in women. The incidence in women is increasing, perhaps due to the use of diuretics in older women with cardiovascular disease. However, there are important links between blood urate and insulin resistance (syndrome X). So musculoskeletal gout may be the tip of a cardiovascular risk 'iceberg'.

Aetiology
Gout is caused by a sustained increase in serum uric acid levels. Uric acid is derived from the breakdown of purine bases, which are components of nucleic acids. It is present in two forms in the body: uric acid and monosodium urate. Synthesis mainly occurs in the liver (Fig. 13.1).

Daily turnover of uric acid is high and approximately two-thirds is renally excreted. Serum levels are related to age, sex, body mass, diet and genetic factors. They are higher in males than in females from puberty until the menopause, when the difference lessens.

Hyperuricaemia is usually due to reduced renal urate excretion, rather than increased production (Fig. 13.2).

Diuretic therapy is probably the commonest cause of gout. Hypoxanthine guanine phosphoribosyltransferase (HGPRT) deficiency is a rare inherited disorder that causes gout in childhood. Complete deficiency of HGPRT occurs in the Lesch–Nyhan syndrome, in which gout is associated with mental retardation, spasticity and self-mutilation.

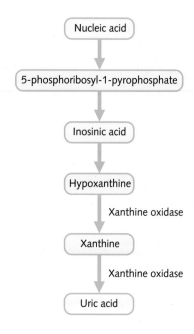

Fig. 13.1 The steps in the synthesis of uric acid.

Some conditions are associated with gout, but do not cause hyperuricaemia. They are shown in Figure 13.3.

Pathology
Prolonged hyperuricaemia leads to the formation of urate crystals. These are deposited in the synovium, other connective tissues and the kidney. Joint inflammation occurs when crystals are shed from deposits within the joint and phagocytosed by polymorphonuclear leucocytes. Urate deposition in the kidney can cause interstitial nephritis, renal stones and acute tubular damage.

Clinical features

Acute gout
Acute gout is extremely painful. It typically presents as a rapidly accelerating monoarthritis, usually affecting the first metatarsophalangeal (MTP) joint (Fig. 13.4). Onset is sudden and symptoms often develop overnight. They include severe pain and

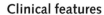

Paediatric hip disorders

Developmental dysplasia of the hip (DDH)
Introduction
Previously called CDH (congenital dislocation of the hip) this disorder is due to failure of normal development of the acetabulum resulting in abnormal hip anatomy. This disorder encompasses the spectrum of disease from a frankly dislocated hip to acetabular dysplasia (in which the slope of the acetabulum is too steep).

Incidence
The incidence is approximately 2 per 1000, although at birth 5–20 per 1000 hips will be unstable. The majority of these settle, stabilize and develop normally without treatment.

Aetiology and pathology
The condition is seven times more common in females. It is also more common in certain races (northern Italy and North American indigenous population).

DDH is associated with:
- Breech presentation.
- Family history.
- Other congenital deformities.

The left side is more commonly affected but the condition is bilateral in 20%.

The acetabulum relies on the presence of the femoral head for normal development. In DDH there is excessive laxity of the joint with a shallow acetabulum (socket) (Fig. 14.2). This allows the femoral head to develop out of the socket, in severe cases forming a false acetabulum (located above the normal one).

Clinical features
The majority are picked up on routine baby check and referred appropriately.

Late-presenting DDH can occur as the child begins to walk. The child will have a limp and shortness of one leg (if unilateral).

The clinical findings of DDH include:
- Loss of abduction.
- Leg length discrepancy.
- Asymmetrical posterior skin crease.

The special tests for dislocated hips are called Barlow's and Ortolani's tests.

Barlow's test
This is an attempt to dislocate a reduced hip.

The examiner's hand is placed so that the child's knee is flexed to 90° and the examiner's thumb is on the medial aspect of the thigh with the middle finger on the trochanter (Fig. 14.3). The child's hip is flexed to 90° and slightly adducted with a slightly downward force applied to try to dislocate the hip. A clunk is felt if positive.

Ortolani's test
This is an attempt to reduce a dislocated hip.

Both hips are examined together. The hand is placed in a similar position and the hip is flexed to 90° and then gently abducted. The test is positive if the hip reduces with a clunk.

Diagnosis and investigation
All babies are screened clinically by examination at birth but unfortunately this is unreliable. At-risk babies with the factors listed above are screened with ultrasound. If there is doubt this investigation can be repeated.

Fig. 14.2 Anatomy of the hip showing (A) normal and (B) pathological hip development.

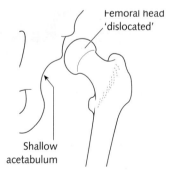

)ulum

al head

Femoral head 'dislocated'

Shallow acetabulum

B   DDH

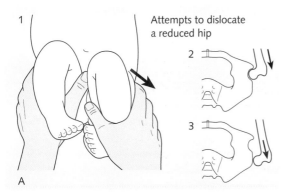

Fig. 14.3 Barlow's test: attempts to dislocate a reduced hip.

An older child should be investigated with X-rays, which once the femoral head has ossified should clearly show if there is a dislocation (Fig. 14.4).

Computed tomography (CT) and magnetic resonance imaging (MRI) scans are now routinely used as part of post-surgery follow-up.

Management
This depends on whether the hip is dislocated and, if so, whether the hip is easily reducible.

Conservative
A Pavlik harness abducts the leg, keeping the hip in joint.

Surgical
If the hip is not reduced, closed or open reduction is performed.

A variety of surgical osteotomies to the pelvis or femur can be used to maintain reduction and 'normalize anatomy'.

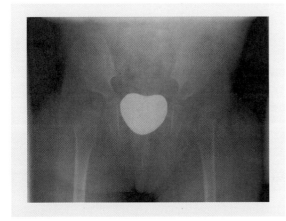

Fig. 14.4 X-ray showing developmental dysplasia of the hip.

Prognosis
The outcome depends upon the degree of dysplasia and whether or not complications such as osteonecrosis develop. Secondary osteoarthritis is common in this group of patients.

Perthes disease
Introduction
This is a rare disease in which there is segmental avascular necrosis of the femoral head.

Incidence
Approximately 1 in 800 are affected.

Aetiology and pathology
Perthes disease is four times more common in boys and is bilateral in 15%. It usually presents between the ages of 4–10.

The condition is associated with:
- Family history.
- Lower socioeconomic groups.
- Low-birthweight children.
- Delayed bone age.

The exact cause of the avascular necrosis is not known.

Following bone death the femoral head changes, initially showing collapse and fragmentation followed by repair and eventual remodelling, which may take many years.

Variable amounts of the head are involved and this has an effect on outcome. Sometimes the head migrates out of the joint (subluxation).

Clinical features
The child (usually a boy) presents with a gradual history of hip or knee pain associated with a limp.

Clinical features will show loss of hip motion, particularly abduction, and there may be fixed deformity. Complete loss of abduction is a worrying sign and may signify subluxation of the hip.

Diagnosis and investigation
Perthes disease in an acutely presenting child could be confused with septic arthritis and therefore blood tests including white cell count (WCC) and inflammatory markers should be performed (all normal in Perthes disease).

A plain X-ray (Fig. 14.5) is the mainstay of diagnosis and is also used to follow the progress of the disease. The features of Perthes on X-ray are:
- Loss of epiphyseal height.
- Increased density.

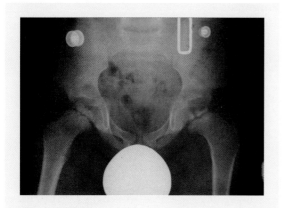

Fig. 14.5 X-ray of Perthes disease.

- Subchondral fracture, partial collapse and fragmentation of the head.
- Abnormal shape and size of femoral head.
- Subluxation.

Treatment

This depends upon the age of the patient and the extent of the disease.

Conservative

A child with an irritable hip may benefit from a period of admission for bed rest and physiotherapy to maintain movement. This applies to most children.

Surgical

Containment of the femoral head may have to be performed surgically. A variety of pelvic or femoral osteotomies can be performed to achieve this.

Prognosis

Young patients with less than 50% involvement of the femoral head have a good prognosis.

Older patients (8 years) with greater than 50% involvement have a poor prognosis, and significant early osteoarthritis is likely.

Slipped upper femoral epiphysis (SUFE)

This condition is a disorder in which there is structural failure through the growth plate of an immature hip.

Incidence

Approximately 3 per 100 000 children are affected.

It is more common in boys than in girls, usually occurring during the early adolescence growth spurt between 11–14 years of age. It presents at a slightly younger age in girls.

Aetiology and pathology

Classically the boy is overweight and has delayed puberty, but this is not always the case.

The exact cause is not known but may relate to failure of the epiphyseal cartilage to mature as the child grows.

The slip results in the epiphysis lying posterior and inferior to the femoral neck.

Approximately 60% are bilateral.

Clinical features

The child presents with groin or knee pain (or both) and a limp. The history can be acute or gradual.

Examination findings reveal an external rotation deformity with limitation of most movements. There may be a slight leg length discrepancy.

Diagnosis and investigation

Diagnosis is based on X-ray changes. An anteroposterior (AP) X-ray is taken, but it is the frog lateral, which most clearly demonstrates the pathology (Fig. 14.6).

 Subtle changes of SUFE can be missed on an AP X-ray. If suspected obtain a frog lateral.

Management
Surgical

All slips should be urgently fixed in situ to prevent further displacement.

Attempts to reduce severe slips are associated with avascular necrosis.

Prognosis

There is a high incidence of secondary degenerative osteoarthritis.

Congenital talipes equinovarus (clubfoot)

Congenital talipes equinovarus (CTEV) encompasses a deformity of the lower limb with calf wasting and the classical inwardly pointing foot.

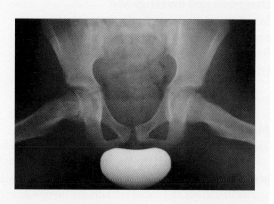

Fig. 14.6 X-ray of SUFE.

Incidence

The incidence is approximately 1 per 1000 live births. Males are affected twice as often as females.

Aetiology and pathology

The exact aetiology is not known but arrest of normal limb bud development in utero may be the cause. Genetic factors play a role with family history being important.

The basic pathology is at the level of the subtalar joint with a cavus deformity (high arch) and metatarsus adductus (Fig. 14.7). The Achilles tendon is also tight, resulting in an equinus deformity.

Associated soft tissue contractures occur on the medial side.

Clinical features

The condition is easily noted at birth as a fixed varus and equinus deformity of the foot. The calf is underdeveloped when compared with the normal side.

The baby should be examined for associated syndromes or conditions.

Diagnosis and investigation

The diagnosis is a clinical one and X-rays are usually taken after initial treatment or surgery.

Management

Conservative

Initial treatment is with serial casting changed weekly for up to 3 months.

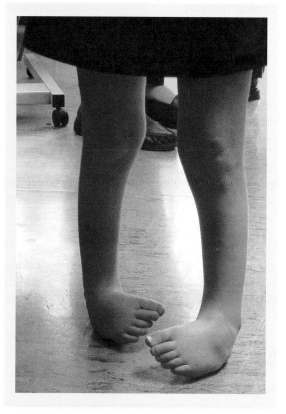

Fig. 14.7 Untreated talipes.

Surgical

Surgery is reserved for those that fail to correct fully or for later recurrence.

Prognosis

The foot and limb will never be normal in terms of appearance but most patients lead a normal life.

Osteogenesis imperfecta

Also known as brittle bone disease, this disorder predisposes to multiple fractures.

Incidence

The condition is rare.

Aetiology and pathology

Osteogenesis imperfecta (OI) is usually inherited as an autosomal dominant condition, although sporadic and recessive cases can occur.

There are four different types of OI.

The primary abnormality is a defect in the synthesis of type 1 collagen.

103

Fig. 14.9 The subtypes of JIA.

complain of pain, whereas a 2-year-old may just be irritable and reluctant to mobilize.

Eye disease
Some forms of JIA can be associated with anterior uveitis. Acute anterior uveitis presents rather obviously with pain and redness of the eye. Chronic anterior uveitis, however, is more insidious and can cause significant visual loss, despite the eye appearing normal to the patient's parents and doctor.

Constitutional symptoms
Fatigue, malaise and other systemic symptoms affect JIA patients, in particular those with systemic onset disease. Growth retardation is an important consequence of prolonged inflammation in childhood.

JIA subtypes
Oligoarticular disease Between one and four joints are affected, commonly in the lower limb. The prognosis for the arthritis is good; many children 'grow out of it'. However, this group of patients has the greatest risk of developing chronic anterior uveitis.

Extended oligoarticular disease Although these patients have involvement of fewer than four joints early in the disease, they gradually develop a polyarthritis after the first 3 months. The outcome is often poor.

Polyarticular disease—rheumatoid factor negative More than four joints are affected from an early stage. This arthritis targets small and large joints and tends to persist into adult life, causing damage and deformity.

Polyarticular disease—rheumatoid factor positive This type of JIA is the equivalent of adult RA. It is seen mainly in teenage girls and frequently has a bad outcome. It may be associated with extra-articular features such as rheumatoid nodules and vasculitis.

Systemic onset disease As the name suggests, this arthritis is characterized by prominent systemic symptoms. It was previously known as Still's disease. Patients present with a swinging fever, plus any of the following features:
- Evanescent rash.
- Hepatomegaly.
- Splenomegaly.
- Anaemia.
- Lymphadenopathy.
- Serositis, especially pericarditis.

The differential diagnosis includes infection and malignancy. Joint involvement may be mild or absent at disease onset.

Enthesitis-related arthritis Inflammation of entheses, e.g. Achilles tendonitis, is a prominent feature. The arthritis is most commonly asymmetrical and affects weight-bearing joints. Enthesitis-related arthritis encompasses juvenile ankylosing spondylitis (AS). A positive family history of AS or related diseases is common and patients are often HLA-B27 positive.

Psoriatic arthritis This is usually oligoarticular and often involves weight-bearing joints. A personal or family history of psoriasis is common.

Investigations
The diagnosis of JIA is essentially clinical. X-rays are helpful in excluding other causes of joint pain, such as infection or malignancy, but are usually normal in early JIA. Blood tests are useful, but not diagnostic. Full blood count may reveal anaemia or thrombocytosis and the erythrocyte sedimentation rate (ESR) and C-reactive protein (CRP) are usually elevated. Serum rheumatoid factor should be measured, especially in teenage girls. It is also important to know if the patient has positive antinuclear antibodies (ANA), as this is associated with an increased risk of uveitis, particularly in oligoarticular disease.

Management

 All children with JIA should be seen by a specialist.

Physiotherapy

Physiotherapy input is vital to maintain mobility and function. Hydrotherapy is commonly used and is popular with children. Splinting is sometimes required to prevent deformity.

Drug treatment

Initial treatment is with regular non-steroidal anti-inflammatory drugs. Disease-modifying therapy with drugs such as methotrexate is used in patients with continued disease activity not responding quickly to other measures. Corticosteroids are avoided where possible, but may be necessary in severe or systemic onset disease. Biological agents, such as the anti-tumour necrosis factor-α drug etanercept, are indicated for seriously ill children with persistent major synovitis or systemic features.

Eye screening

Children with some types of JIA should have their eyes examined regularly by an ophthalmologist. Early signs of chronic anterior uveitis can only be seen on slit-lamp examination. The risk is highest in the ANA-positive oligoarticular group. Screening is not needed in enthesitis-related arthritis or older children with positive rheumatoid factors and adult-type disease.

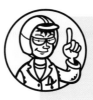

Eye screening is particularly important in young children with JIA, as they do not reliably report visual disturbance to their parents.

- What factors increase the likelihood of having a child with developmental dysplasia of the hip (DDH)?
- What is the incidence of DDH?
- What are the pathological features of DDH?
- What investigations are performed in DDH, at what age and why?
- What treatment options are there?
- Who is more likely to get Perthes disease?
- What are the X-ray features of Perthes disease? slipped upper femoral epiphysis (SUFE)?
- What are the basic principles of treatment in Perthes disease?
- How common is SUFE?
- At what age do the three childhood hip conditions usually present?
- What is the usual presentation of Perthes disease? SUFE?
- What is the current treatment for SUFE?
- When does congenital talipes equinovarus (CTEV) present?
- What are the pathological features of CTEV?
- How do you manage CTEV?
- What is the underlying problem in osteogenesis imperfecta (OI)?
- Outline basic management of OI?
- What is osteochondritis?
- What is Osgood–Schlatter disease and how do you treat it?

Further reading

Cassidy, Petty 2001 Textbook of Paediatric Rheumatology. Saunders
Dandy D J 1998 Essentials of orthopaedics and trauma, 3rd edn. Churchill Livingstone, London
Miller M D 2000 Review of orthopaedics, 3rd edn. WB Saunders, Philadelphia

Solomon L, Warwick D, Nayagan D (eds) 2001 Apley's system of orthopaedics and fractures, 8th edn. Hodder Arnold, London
Orthoteers website: http://www.orthoteers.co.uk

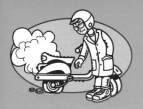

15. Fractures

In this chapter we will discuss the basic principles of managing fractures. It is not the intention of this book to be an extensive guide for each individual fracture nor will we cover advanced trauma life support (ATLS) and the management of a multiply injured patient.

Incidence
Fractures are very common and most of us will have at least one during a lifetime. They occur in peaks during childhood, young adult life and again in the elderly when osteoporosis has weakened bony structure (see Ch. 12).

Pathology and aetiology
Fractures can occur through normal bone if the force applied is large enough, or be pathological and occur through abnormal or diseased bone. Figure 15.1 shows the causes of pathological fractures.

In children the fracture may occur through the growth plate, and these injuries are classified as shown in Figure 15.2.

The mechanism of injury dictates the fracture pattern. A twisting injury produces a spiral fracture and a direct blow from the side a transverse or oblique fracture. See Figure 15.3.

As the force applied increases so does the severity of injury; a patient falling 50 feet will have

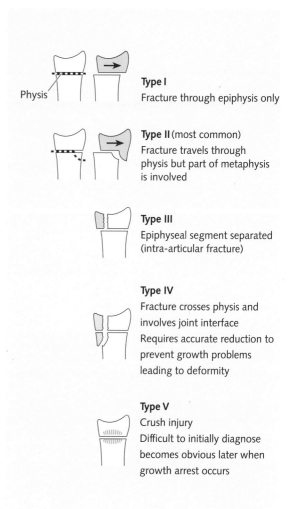

Type I
Fracture through epiphysis only

Type II (most common)
Fracture travels through physis but part of metaphysis is involved

Type III
Epiphyseal segment separated (intra-articular fracture)

Type IV
Fracture crosses physis and involves joint interface
Requires accurate reduction to prevent growth problems leading to deformity

Type V
Crush injury
Difficult to initially diagnose becomes obvious later when growth arrest occurs

Fig. 15.2 The Salter–Harris classification of fractures of the growth plate (physeal fractures).

Underlying causes in pathological fractures
Osteoporosis
Tumours • Benign • Malignant
Paget's disease
Metabolic bone disease • Osteomalacia/rickets • Hyperparathyroidism • Osteogenesis imperfecta
Other malignancy • Lymphoma • Myeloma
Rheumatoid arthritis
Infection

Fig. 15.1 Underlying causes in pathological fractures.

more serious injuries than one twisting an ankle. A bone fails because the load exceeds its strength.

Fractures can be open (associated with a wound) (Fig. 15.4) or closed (skin intact). Open fractures allow contamination of the bone ends, predisposing to deep bony infection (see Ch. 16).

Injuries may also involve the joint surface (intra-articular) or the bone may be in lots of pieces (multi-fragmentary).

Fig. 15.3 Fracture patterns.

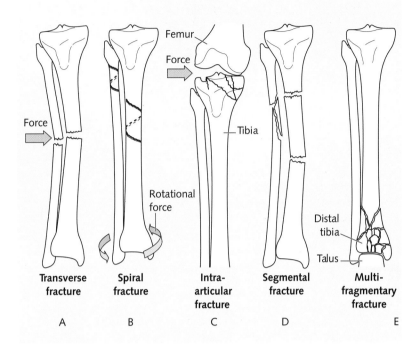

Transverse fracture	Spiral fracture	Intra-articular fracture	Segmental fracture	Multi-fragmentary fracture
A	B	C	D	E

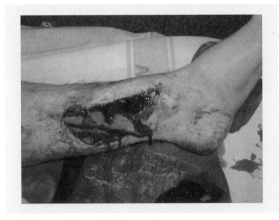

Fig. 15.4 An open tibial fracture.

A segmental fracture occurs in the diaphysis (shaft) at two levels, leaving a 'floating segment'.

When concentrating on the bone it is easy to forget the soft tissues surrounding the bone. It is the soft tissues that will eventually provide a healing environment via blood vessel attachment to the injured bone.

Clinical features

The patient almost always gives a clear history of an injury such as falling off a slide, playing football or a simple trip. Difficulty can arise if the patient cannot give a history (e.g. because of dementia), in which case the history may be obtained from the carer or a relative but sometimes there is no history of a fall.

Patients will complain of severe pain and they may have noticed a deformity (e.g. 'my ankle pointed the wrong way doctor').

The whole patient should be examined for associated injuries and then the injured limb.

The affected limb will be swollen and bruised with significant tenderness to palpation. Fracture crepitus can be felt and heard on movement but this is cruel and unnecessary (plus moving the fracture excessively may further damage soft tissues).

It is very important to note:

- Skin condition (i.e. open or closed, but also note blisters and abrasions).
- Peripheral nerve function—any weakness or numbness of the hand or foot.
- Distal vascular status—assess peripheral pulse and perfusion.

Compare the abnormal with the normal limb.

The patient may also have a clinical deformity associated with a particular fracture such as a dinner fork deformity in Colles' fracture.

Patients with suspected spinal injuries need to be log-rolled for examination and a full peripheral nervous system examination performed.

Diagnosis and investigation

X-rays should be taken in two planes at 90° to each other (anteroposterior (AP) and lateral) to give accurate information on the suspected fractured bone (Fig. 15.5). If there may be an associated joint injury, X-rays of the joint are needed. Special views are taken for certain fractures (e.g. scaphoid views).

Computed tomography (CT) scans are helpful to plan surgery in very severe multi-fragmentary intra-articular fractures.

Magnetic resonance imaging (MRI) or isotope bone scans are occasionally used to diagnose a fracture where doubt exists. MRI is also useful in the follow-up of certain fractures to look for avascular necrosis.

Describing fractures

This is something all medical students are very bad at!

Follow the steps outlined below:
- Name and age of patient, and date of X-ray.
- Remember **ABC**.
- **A** is for Adequacy and Alignment (Is the film rotated? Of acceptable quality, i.e. too light or too dark?).
- **B** is for Bone.
  - State which bone, e.g. tibia.
  - Where in the bone, i.e. metaphysis/diaphysis/epiphysis.
  - Fracture pattern; transverse, oblique, spiral, segmental, multi-fragmentary.
  - Deformity (Fig. 15.6):
    —displacement
    —angulation
    —shortening
    —rotation (can be difficult to appreciate unless the joints above and below are seen)
  - Joint: intra-articular, dislocation.
- **C** is for soft tissues: look for air (may indicate an open fracture), swelling or joint fluid.

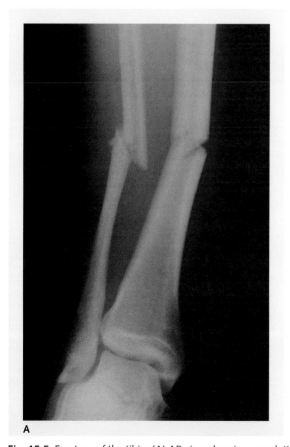

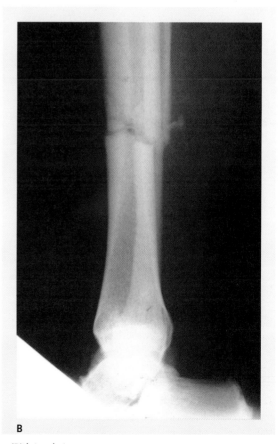

Fig. 15.5 Fracture of the tibia: (A) AP view showing angulation; (B) lateral view.

Remember to add important clinical features when describing the fracture:
- general condition of patient
- skin (open or closed)
- neurovascular status.

Management

The basic principles for the treatment of any fracture are:

- Reduction of any deformity (displacement, angulation, rotation), i.e. put the bones back into the correct place.
- Stabilization (maintain reduction until healing occurs).
- Rehabilitation (rehabilitate the limb and the person back to normality).

Reduction

Reduction can be performed open or closed.

- Closed reduction is performed by manipulating the fracture into position. A Colles' fracture is a good example of a fracture treated with closed reduction.
- Open reduction is performed in the operating theatre and involves a surgical procedure to open up the fracture site and accurately reduce the bones under direct vision.

Intra-articular fractures are treated with open reduction so that the joint can be accurately reduced, minimizing the risk of secondary osteoarthritis.

Stabilization

The fracture can be stabilized by conservative or operative treatment. The choice of treatment depends on the bone and fracture characteristics.

Internal fixation allows early mobilization and prevents displacement but there are risks of surgery.

Plaster casts avoid the risk of surgery but there is a chance the fracture will re-displace, and deformity may result if malunion occurs.

Conservative

A plaster of Paris cast is the most common form of conservative treatment used.

Fig. 15.6 Deformity associated with fractures.

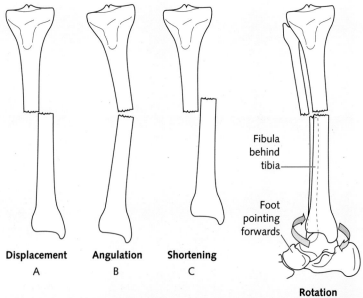

Displacement
A

Angulation
B

Shortening
C

Fibula behind tibia

Foot pointing forwards

Rotation
D

The cast should immobilize the joint above and below the fracture and be moulded into position in order to minimize the position 'slipping' in a cast.

Traction used to be widespread on orthopaedic wards but is rarely used nowadays. Traction uses weight to pull fracture fragments into alignment and maintain reduction. The disadvantage of traction is the prolonged treatment with risks of bedsores, deep vein thrombosis (DVT) and chest complications.

Operative

Operative treatment is always required for open fractures and displaced intra-articular fractures. Other fractures may be treated in this way, particularly if they are unstable.

There are several different methods of surgical stabilization (Fig. 15.7):

1. Percutaneous wiring: commonly performed at the wrist. Wires are passed across the fracture site to hold the bone reduced. They are removed at 4–6 weeks.
2. Internal fixation: a plate and screws hold the fracture rigidly.
3. Intramedullary nail: a nail is passed in the medullary cavity and locked at both ends. This is commonly used in the tibia and femur.

4. External fixation: pins or wires inserted into the bone are held by a 'frame' externally.

Rehabilitation

Following healing, or if the fracture is stable, the limb can be mobilized and range of movement exercises begun. The physiotherapist may need to instruct the patient in the use of crutches for restricted weight bearing.

Rehabilitation of the limb may often take as much time as the fracture took to heal.

Following a hip fracture elderly patients require intensive input from physiotherapy, occupational therapy and social workers in order to become self-caring and safe prior to discharge.

Complications of fractures

Any complication can be local or general; and immediate, early or late.

Immediate
Local

Initial displacement can cause the skin to tear resulting in an open fracture. Fracture fragments may press on nerves producing a nerve palsy (common in the humerus, resulting in radial nerve palsy) or blood vessels producing ischaemia (e.g. femur—popliteal vessels). See Figure 15.8.

Fig. 15.7 Methods of surgical stabilization of fractures.

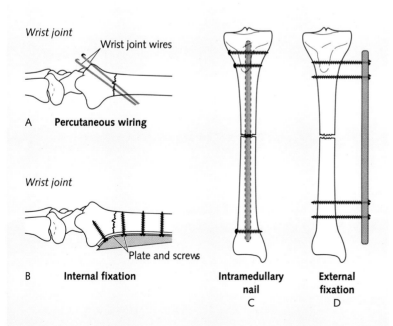

A **Percutaneous wiring**
Wrist joint
Wrist joint wires

B **Internal fixation**
Wrist joint
Plate and screws

C **Intramedullary nail**

D **External fixation**

Very occasionally nerves and blood vessels are torn completely and repair is needed.

General

Haemorrhage from fractures can be excessive if open or if there is more than one fracture. Hypovolaemic shock may result.

Early
Local

Compartment syndrome This is an important complication and results from excessive pressure developing in closed fascial muscle compartments. Following a fracture, swelling can cause the blood supply to the muscle to be impaired. This occurs at the level of small vessels, and peripheral pulses are usually still present. The patient will complain of excessive pain (more than normal) and pain on passive movement of the digits is demonstrated. Paraesthesia may be present. The diagnosis can be confirmed with pressure monitoring, and if so, surgical fasciotomy (release of compartments) should be performed.

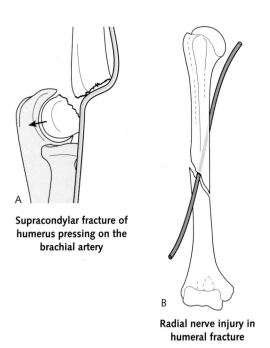

A **Supracondylar fracture of humerus pressing on the brachial artery**

B **Radial nerve injury in humeral fracture**

Fig. 15.8 Neurovascular complications of fractures.

Infection This can occur early or late following operative stabilization or open fracture. See Chapter 16.

Reflex sympathetic dystrophy This unusual condition can occur after any injury or operation. The exact cause is not known but is thought to relate to the sympathetic nervous system.

Usually the upper limb is affected. The patient has red, swollen shiny fingers with excessive joint stiffness. Atypical pain is also a feature. Physiotherapy is the mainstay of this difficult condition.

General

Deep vein thrombosis DVT can occur after any lower limb injury. Prevention in the form of mechanical (foot pumps, graduated compression stockings) or chemical (heparin, aspirin) agents is routinely used.

Diagnosis is often difficult as the limb will be swollen and may be painful because of the injury. If in doubt obtain a duplex scan or venogram. Some at-risk patients are treated prophylactically with warfarin.

Fat embolus This important condition is common after long bone fractures (particularly of the femur) and occurs due to fat entering the circulation and embolizing to the lungs. The condition occurs because the medullary canal of long bones contain fat. Early stabilization of fractures reduces the risk.

The patient presents with shortness of breath, petechial haemorrhages and sometimes confusion from low circulating Po_2 usually 2–3 days after injury.

This condition is potentially very serious and may lead on to acute adult respiratory failure (ARDS), which can be fatal.

Treatment is supportive with oxygen and fluids. Transfer to a high-dependency unit is advised.

Late
Delayed union/non-union

Some fractures are slow to unite or fail to do so despite adequate treatment. Certain fractures (e.g. of the tibia) are more prone to this and it is more likely if the initial injury was high energy or complicated by compartment syndrome. Further surgery may be required to encourage the bone to heal.

Malunion

The fracture heals but in an abnormal position. This is usually due to inadequate stabilization of the fracture. The resulting deformity may reduce movement in an associated joint and predisposes to late arthritis.

Osteoarthritis

Osteoarthritis, which is discussed in Chapter 8, is more common after intra-articular fractures.

Stiffness

Prolonged immobilization can result in severe joint stiffness.

Contracture

Untreated compartment syndrome or vascular complication can result in contracture. Volkmann's ischaemic contracture is an example.

Growth disturbance

Fractures occurring through the growth plate can cause deformity if the growth arrest is partial (i.e. one side of the limb grows, the other does not) or shortness of the limb if complete. Treatment of such problems is complex.

- Who gets fractures?
- What conditions predispose to pathological fractures?
- How can you group fractures?
- Describe the fracture shown in Figure 15.5.
- What are the clinical features of a broken bone?
- What investigations can you perform to confirm a fracture?
- What are the basic principles of fracture treatment?
- How many different types of operative treatment are there?
- Which fractures should always be treated with operative fixation?
- What conservative methods of treatment are there?
- What are the common complications of fractures?
- What is fat embolus and when does it present?

Further reading

Charnley J 1999 The closed treatment of common fractures, new Golden Jubilee edn. Colt Books, Cambridge (*only £15 and gives an excellent practical account of plaster and traction techniques*)
Dandy D J 1998 Essentials of orthopaedics and trauma, 3rd edn. Churchill Livingstone, London

Miller M D 2000 Review of orthopaedics, 3rd edn. WB Saunders, Philadelphia
Solomon L, Warwick D, Nayagan D (eds) 2001 Apley's system of orthopaedics and fractures, 8th edn. Hodder Arnold, London
Orthoteers website: http://www.orthoteers.co.uk

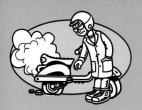

16. Infection of Bones and Joints

Introduction

Bone and joint infection has become much less common in western society over the last century. This is explained by increasing use of antibiotics and the general improvement in nutrition and health of the population as a whole.

Infection does still occur and needs to be recognized and treated promptly to avoid potentially serious complications.

In this chapter we will talk about osteomyelitis (infection in bone) and septic arthritis (infection in a joint).

In order for you to have an understanding of why infection develops in bone we must revise some simple anatomy (Fig. 16.1).

Blood supply to bone is from the endosteum and periosteum.

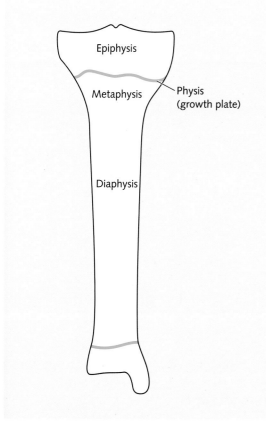

Fig. 16.1 Basic anatomy of a bone.

Osteomyelitis

Infection of bone can be caused by direct inoculation (exogenous) or blood-borne bacteria (haematogenous).

In childhood or adolescence osteomyelitis is usually caused by haematogenous spread of bacteria. In adults the source is more likely to be exogenous, most commonly due to infection developing after surgery or after injury (particularly in the case of an open fracture).

Incidence

Osteomyelitis is now uncommon.

Aetiology and pathology

In children there is often a history of preceding trauma, which may predispose the limb to infection. The most common infecting organism overall is *Staphylococcus aureus*, but streptococcal (neonates particularly) and Gram-negative infections can also occur. If unusual organisms are present consider specific predisposing factors as listed in Figure 16.3, for example patients with AIDS can get fungal infections.

The three most common causes of osteomyelitis are:
- Post-trauma osteomyelitis.
- Post-surgery osteomyelitis.
- Acute haematogenous osteomyelitis.

Post-trauma osteomyelitis

An open fracture means the skin is broken allowing bacteria direct access to the bony surfaces. Large dirty wounds associated with high-energy injuries are more likely to result in post-trauma osteomyelitis. Urgent surgical debridement and lavage are required in order to remove contaminated material and dead bone. Inadequate or delayed surgery often leads to osteomyelitis due to bacteria being harboured within dead bone. In these circumstances the fracture will often fail to unite.

Post-surgery osteomyelitis

Many surgical procedures in orthopaedics involve using implants such as hip replacements or plates and screws. These 'foreign bodies' can harbour infection if at the time of surgery bacteria are introduced. For this reason orthopaedic surgeons are strict about aseptic techniques in the operating theatre and use antibiotics as prophylaxis. Despite this, infection does still occur and may spread around the implant, devitalizing bone.

Acute haematogenous osteomyelitis

This form of osteomyelitis is usually seen in children and may develop spontaneously.

The pathogenesis of acute haematogenous osteomyelitis is as follows (Fig. 16.2):

1. Trauma to affected limb.
2. A bacteraemia that settles in the metaphysis of a long bone.
3. The metaphysis has a good blood supply but is thought to have very few phagocytic cells capable of fighting infection, therefore allowing the infection to develop.
4. Inflammation and pus formation within the bone.
5. Pus escapes through small holes in bone (harversian canals) to form a subperiosteal abscess.
6. Pus is now present on both sides of the bone, causing this part of the bone to die.

7. Dead bone now called the *sequestrum* harbours infection.
8. Periosteal new bone called *involucrum* forms as the body tries to fight the infection.
9. In older children the *physis* (growth plate) acts as a barrier, preventing further spread of infection.
10. In neonates and infants spread can occur across the physis via the epiphyseal artery.
11. In some joints the capsule extends down to the metaphysis. If pus escapes here, then septic arthritis will result.

Acute osteomyelitis can easily become chronic if the sequestrum is neglected or not completely excised at surgery.

Other conditions associated with osteomyelitis

The above three causes of osteomyelitis are the most common but it also occurs in the other conditions listed in Figure 16.3.

Sadly we are now seeing more and more cases of bone and joint infection in intravenous drug users. When you consider that these patients are often malnourished, immunosuppressed (possibly HIV positive), frequently inject themselves deeply with

Fig. 16.2 Sequence of events in osteomyelitis. The primary focus of infection (A) has spread through bone, causing the death of cortical bone and formation of a subperiosteal abscess (B). Infection can spread into the joint (C) causing septic arthritis. Death of a segment of bone (sequestrum) occurs (D), and the area is surrounded by new subperiosteal bone (involucrum).

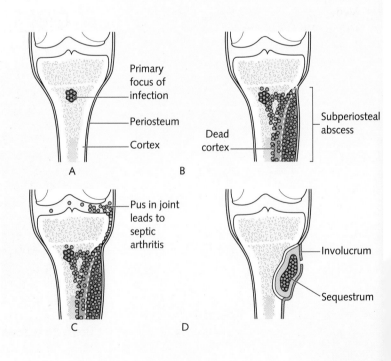

Conditions associated with osteomyelitis	
Congenital	**Acquired**
Sickle cell disease	Diabetes
Haemophilia	Renal failure
	Intravenous drug use
	Malnutrition
	Immunosuppression
	HIV/AIDS

Fig. 16.3 Conditions associated with osteomyelitis.

dirty needles and often neglect small abscesses it is not difficult to understand why.

Clinical features

Acute osteomyelitis causes pain, fever and loss of funtion (often a limp if the lower limb is involved).

It is more common in the tibia and femur. The limb will be tender to palpate, erythematous and possibly swollen.

At the extremes of age (neonate, infant or elderly) the symptoms and signs are often non-specific (such as general malaise). These patients can be seriously ill and it can be extremely difficult to pinpoint the exact site of the problem.

Occasionally a patient presents with multiple sites affected or there may be another focus of infection which has then spread from or to bone, for example infective endocarditis. This is called seeding of infection.

In post-surgery and post-trauma osteomyelitis the wound will be painful, red and inflamed. Normally once postoperative pain has settled, patients are comfortable and can mobilize without pain. If pain persists or increases, infection is a possible cause. Eventually wounds will break down and discharge. If left untreated a sinus will result.

A limb with chronic osteomyelitis will be swollen and have thickened 'woody' skin. Here the focus of infection remains within the bone as a sequestrum and the infection remains quiet for a period of time (can be many years) and then flares up unexpectedly, often producing as abscess. A chronic discharging sinus can result.

Diagnosis and investigation

The diagnosis may be obvious on clinical features, particularly if the history reveals a clear predisposing factor.

A raised white cell count (WCC), erythrocyte sedimentation rate (ESR) and C-reactive protein (CRP) will be present on blood tests.

Initially X-rays will be normal, but after 10 days, features of lysis, periosteal elevation and new bone formation are seen. Later the sequestrum may be seen as a sclerotic area. A Brodie's abscess may be seen in the distal femur (Fig. 16.4).

Early osteomyelitis can be detected before X-ray changes, using bone scanning (shows increased uptake) or magnetic resonance imaging (MRI).

It is very important to send microbiology specimens such as blood cultures prior to starting antibiotics.

Management
Conservative

The patient needs adequate analgesia, splintage of the affected limb and appropriate antibiotics. Consultation with the microbiologist is advisable.

As the majority of infections are with *Staph. aureus*, flucloxacillin and fusidic acid are usually the first-line antibiotics given initially intravenously for 6 weeks.

Antibiotic-resistant strains such as MRSA are becoming more prevalent and if suspected then

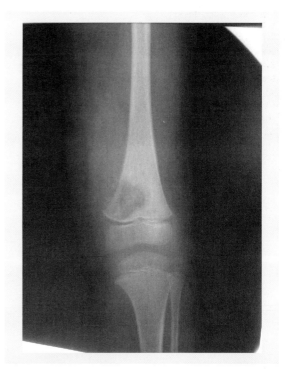

Fig. 16.4 Brodie's abscess.

vancomycin is usually the antibiotic of choice (consult a microbiologist).

Provided the patient does not have an abscess or dead bone present, then antibiotics will suffice.

Surgical

If an abscess is present this should be drained surgically. Dead bone, the sequestrum, needs to be removed.

In a chronic case if the patient and surgeon decide to attempt to cure the infection, extensive surgery is required to remove the implant and all infected bone. Techniques for doing this vary depending on the extent of involvement and the site.

It is possible to simply treat the 'flare-ups' and suppress the infection with antibiotics when required.

Complications

Complications occur if:
- Osteomyelitis persists.
- The physis is damaged, leading to growth disturbance and deformity.
- The infection spreads to the joint, causing septic arthritis.

Prognosis

For acute osteomyelitis the outcome is good and the majority make a full recovery provided none of the above complications occur. In chronic cases following surgery or trauma many surgical procedures are often required and amputation is not an uncommon outcome.

Septic arthritis

Septic arthritis is infection within a synovial joint.

Incidence

The condition is uncommon, but is seen more often in children, young adults and the elderly. It is more common in the developing world and in patients with a predisposing factor. In children, it is less common than osteomyelitis.

Aetiology and pathology

Infection reaches a joint via the haematogenous route, direct spread from the metaphysis or penetrating trauma/surgery. Associated conditions are similar to those for acute osteomyelitis (see

Fig. 16.3) with the addition of rheumatoid arthritis and crystal arthropathy.

Certain organisms are more common at different ages. *Haemophilus influenzae* used to be the most common infecting organism in infants prior to the introduction of the vaccination programme. In young sexually active adults the most likely infecting organism is *Neisseria gonorrhoeae*.

In haematogenous septic arthritis the bacterium settles in the synovium, which may be inflamed due to trauma or disease. Proliferation of bacteria causes an inflammatory response by the host with numerous leucocytes migrating into the joint. The variety of enzymes and breakdown products produced damages the delicate articular cartilage very quickly (within hours) and if left unchecked permanent damage will ensue (Fig. 16.5).

Clinical features

The patient will have an acutely hot swollen joint with a fever and be systemically unwell. An infant or young child will be distressed, unwell and difficult to assess! There may be a history of recent infection such as otitis media.

Septic arthritis is more common in the hip and knee but can present in the shoulder, elbow and wrist.

Any movement at all causes intense pain, and weight bearing will not be tolerated. If the joint is superficial an effusion is palpable.

In neonates and infants the diagnosis may be less obvious, particularly if the joint is deeply situated such as the hip. These patients may be seriously ill.

Patients with an infected joint will not let you put the joint through a passive range of movement. It is too painful!

Diagnosis and investigation
- WCC, CRP and ESR will be raised.
- X-rays will be normal and are often unnecessary.
- If available, ultrasound scanning is useful to see if there is a joint effusion where the hip is the suspicious joint.
- If the joint aspirate is cloudy, it is sent for urgent Gram stain, culture and examination for crystals.

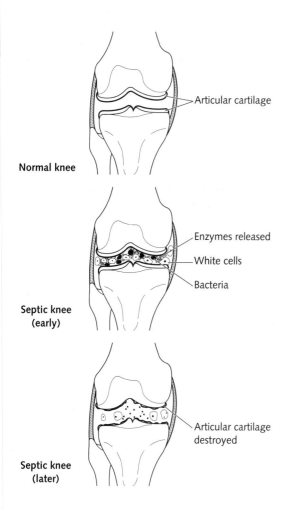

Normal knee

Septic knee
(early)

Articular cartilage

Enzymes released

White cells

Bacteria

Septic knee
(later)

Articular cartilage
destroyed

Fig. 16.5 Sequence of events in septic arthritis.

Management
Conservative
Relieve pain by giving analgesia and splinting the limb. Give appropriate antibiotics as directed by the microbiologist depending on the age of the patient and any predisposing illness.

Surgical
Unlike in osteomyelitis the treatment of septic arthritis is always surgical drainage. This should be done as an emergency to limit the damage to the joint cartilage.

Complications
- Seeding of infection can occur to the spine or other organs.
- Recurrence of infection.
- Joint destruction with long-term arthritis or even anklyosis (bony fusion across the joint).
- Avascular necrosis (particularly in the hip).

Prognosis
If treated promptly, prognosis is good, but if joint destruction occurs it is very poor.

Tuberculosis

Incidence
Tuberculosis (TB) is common in global terms and causes significant morbidity and mortality in Africa and Asia.

TB is making a 'comeback' in the UK with over 10 000 cases per year, mainly in the Asian community.

Aetiology and pathology
TB is due to *Mycobacterium tuberculosis* or *Mycobacterium bovis* infection.

Histologically the classical appearance is of caeseating necrosis.

Musculoskeletal tuberculosis results when primary TB (lung) becomes widespread or when later reactivation or reinfection occurs (immunosuppressed patients).

Clinical features
Patients have general symptoms of ill-health such as malaise, weight loss, cough and loss of appetite. The most common musculoskeletal sites affected by TB are the spine, hip and knee.

Unlike other orthopaedic infections, TB presents with gradual symptoms of pain and may be initially diagnosed as osteoarthritis or inflammatory arthritis.

Diagnosis and investigation
The two commonest tests are the Mantoux and Heaf tests, which are skin hypersensitivity tests.

For confirmation, large samples of bone or synovial fluid are required which need to be cultured for a prolonged period (6 weeks).

If mycobacterial infection is suspected, samples should be submitted to a Ziehl–Neelsen stain and the mycobacteria appear as red acid–alcohol-fast organisms.

X-rays show variable amounts of joint destruction with periarticular osteopenia.

Management

There is no specific treatment for fibromyalgia. Quality of life for most patients remains poor. The following treatment strategies may help.

Education

- Informs patients about the condition.
- Reassures them that they do not have a destructive arthritis or underlying malignancy.
- Emphasizes that they will not harm their joints by exercising.

Cognitive behavioural therapy

This encourages patients to develop mechanisms to cope with their symptoms.

Drug therapy

Low-dose amitriptyline can help sleep, fatigue and pain.

Physiotherapy

A graded aerobic exercise regime may have some benefit.

Fig. 17.3 The 'tender points' of fibromyalgia.

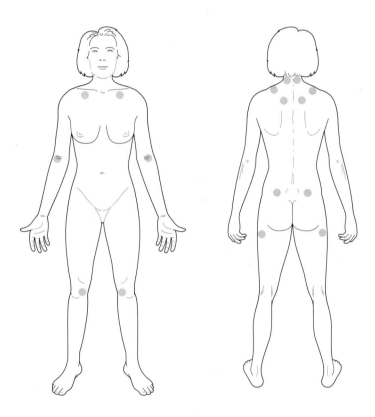

- List the common symptoms of fibromyalgia.
- What are the common sites of tissue tenderness?
- Discuss strategies employed in the management of patients with fibromyalgia.

Further reading

Arthritis Research Campaign patient information leaflet

Goldenberg D L 2003 Fibromyalgia and related syndrome. In: Hochberg et al (eds) *Rheumatology*, 3rd edn. Mosby, London, p 701-712

Ryan S Fibromyalgia. In : *ABC of Rheumatology*, 3rd edn. BMJ Books, London

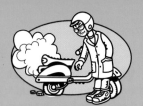

Orthopaedic operations are very common and this chapter outlines the principles of surgery.

Sterility

Infection is the major concern in elective orthopaedic surgery. For example, if a joint replacement becomes infected, simple measures such as antibiotics and abscess drainage will not eradicate the infection. The patient may be worse off than before surgery and require lengthy hospital stays with extensive further surgery and significant risks.

The risk of infection is minimized by the following preoperative, perioperative and postoperative factors.

Preoperative factors

- Cleaning the skin.
- Avoidance of concurrent infection (e.g. urinary tract infection).
- Preoperative antibiotics.
- A healthy, well-nourished patient.

Perioperative factors

- Clean laminar airflow theatre (air is specially filtered).
- Adequate skin preparation and impervious exclusion drapes.
- Exhaust suits (enclosed clothing with air evacuation to prevent skin contaminants falling onto the wound).
- Sterile instruments and prostheses.
- Careful surgical technique (including haemostasis).

Postoperative factors

- Wound dressing.
- Prophylactic antibiotics for possible bacteraemia (e.g. during catheterization).

Operations

There are several things a surgeon can do for a painful joint.

Joint debridement

A diseased joint can be debrided surgically in an attempt to improve range of movement or to reduce symptoms such as pain and swelling.

Debridement means removing diseased tissue. Osteophytes are often removed in osteoarthritis but debriding a joint does not cure or stop the progression of the disease process.

Examples of joints where debridement is performed include the first metatarsophalangeal (MTP) joint in hallux rigidus. See Figure 18.1.

Arthroscopy

'Keyhole surgery' techniques have become routine in recent years.

In the past, arthroscopy was seen as a diagnostic procedure but now a number of operations are possible by purely arthroscopic means. Examples are

First metatarsophalangeal joint arthritis

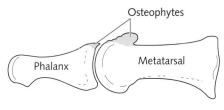

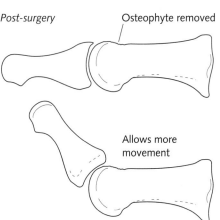

Fig. **18.1** Joint debridement.

It is also possible to lengthen bones gradually with external fixation usually in the form of circular frames with a variety of hinges and movable rods. See Figure 18.7.

Operations for rheumatoid arthritis

In Chapter 9 there is a lot of information about the diagnosis and medical treatment of rheumatoid arthritis but the majority of patients with rheumatoid disease will have surgery at some stage and some have multiple operations (you may come across a patient with shoulders, elbows, hips and knees replaced, and both wrists and ankles fused!).

Synovectomy

The aim of this operation is to remove the synovial lining of the diseased joint or the tenosynovium around tendons. It is only practical to perform this operation when the disease is in the relatively early stages and the patient has chronic synovitis. This has three possible beneficial effects:

1. reduction of swelling
2. slowing of disease progression
3. prevention of tendon rupture.

Unfortunately it is impossible to remove the whole synovium with synovectomy, and symptoms often return. This procedure is usually performed around the wrist.

Operations commonly performed on rheumatoid patients are shown in Figure 18.8.

Fig. 18.7 Deformity correction with frames. (A) The use of an external fixator 'frame' to achieve gradual correction of a deformity over several weeks. Note that the frame is also bent but straightens out as the bone is corrected. (B) Ilizarov frame on a fractured tibia.

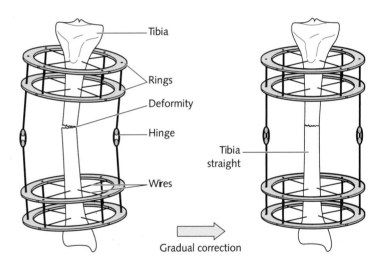

A

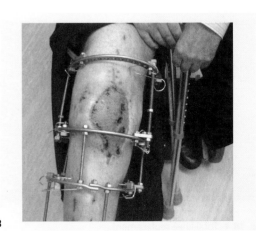

B

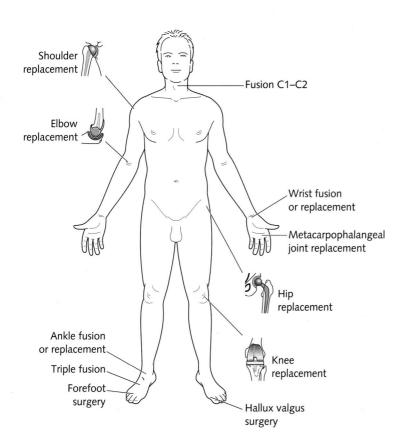

Fig. 18.8 Common operations for rheumatoid patients.

Shoulder replacement

Elbow replacement

Fusion C1–C2

Wrist fusion or replacement

Metacarpophalangeal joint replacement

Hip replacement

Ankle fusion or replacement

Triple fusion

Forefoot surgery

Knee replacement

Hallux valgus surgery

- What factors can reduce the risks of infection in orthopaedics?
- What types of surgery can be performed on a joint?
- What is an osteotomy? Think of an example.
- Which joints are commonly examined using arthroscopy?
- Which joints are commonly replaced?
- Where is fusion more commonly performed?
- Write a list of operations for rheumatoid arthritis.

Further reading

Canale S T 2003 Campbell's operative orthopaedics, 10th edn. Mosby, St Louis, vols 1–4

Fitzgerald R H, Kaufer H, Malkani A (eds) 2002 Orthopaedics. Mosby, Philadelphia

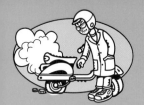

19. Pre and Postoperative Care

Orthopaedics is a surgical speciality and one of the tasks of a junior doctor is to assess patients prior to surgery and look after them postoperatively.

Any surgical procedure has risks and complications, and knowledge of these helps minimize and prevent them.

Patients now need to be made aware of these important complications before informed consent is obtained.

Complications are divided into:
- Local (specific to that operation), and
- general (common to any operation).

We further subdivide complication on the basis of the time that has elapsed after surgery, into:
- Immediate (within 24 hours).
- Early (days/weeks).
- Late (months/years).

Preoperative assessment

Complications can be minimized by careful preoperative preparation. Any concurrent medical problems need to be stabilized and new conditions identified, investigated and treated appropriately.

Nowadays elective patients are seen a few weeks before surgery in the preoperative assessment clinic. The following should be recorded.

General
- Observations (BP, pulse, temperature): the patient may have undiagnosed atrial fibrillation (AF) or hypertension.
- History including past medical history and drug history: the patient may be on warfarin and will need this to be stopped prior to surgery and may need admission for intravenous heparin.
- Detailed systemic enquiry: the patient may have shortness of breath on exertion and chest pain (angina). Such a patient following investigation may even go on to have coronary bypass surgery prior to the orthopaedic operation.
- Examination: e.g. the patient may have a heart murmur.
- Blood tests (unnecessary in young, fit patients for simple surgery): full blood count (FBC), glucose,

urea and electrolytes (U&E), liver function tests (LFTs) and clotting screen. Sickle cell test for patients of Afro-Caribbean origin. Arterial blood gases may be required if the patient has chest disease.
- Blood can be grouped and saved and cross-matched if significant blood loss is expected.
- Urinalysis for diabetes mellitus or urinary tract infection (UTI). If a patient has an UTI, it should be treated prior to any orthopaedic operation.
- Electrocardiogram (ECG) and chest X-ray (if indicated).
- Further investigations should be ordered if required, e.g. cardiac echo in aortic stenosis.

Informed consent should be taken by a surgeon capable of performing the operation so that particular risks and expectations can be explained to the patient. This means the pre-registration House Officer is not the best person for the job!

Local
The patient should be asked if the limb is still painful because the surgery may be unnecessary.

The limb is examined.

Note skin condition (there may be a rash or skin breakdown over the operation site), pulses, range of movement and look for any distal infection. For example, a knee replacement procedure should not be carried out in a patient with an infected ingrowing toenail.

Immediate preoperative care

Additional monitoring such as an arterial line and central venous line can be inserted in the anaesthetic room for patients expected to have a complicated anaesthetic.

A urinary catheter is important to assess fluid balance in patients who may lose significant amounts of blood.

Intravenous antibiotics and deep vein thrombosis (DVT) prophylaxis are also given if necessary.

As soon as possible, physiotherapy is encouraged, to mobilize the limb.

Basic postoperative care

General

Patients are taken to recovery until fully awake, then transferred to a high-dependency unit (HDU) or the ward.

Regular recordings are made of BP, pulse and oxygen saturation.

Adequate pain relief is very important.

Check sensation, perfusion, pulses and function of digits distal to the operative field.

After major surgery requiring an inpatient stay, patients will need:
- FBC and U&E checked the day after surgery.
- X-rays of the joint operated upon.

Once patients are well, every effort is made to mobilize them and encourage early safe discharge. DVT prophylaxis is continued until patients are mobile.

A multidisciplinary approach is needed to achieve this, with physiotherapy, occupational therapy, social workers, nursing staff and sometimes physicians having input.

Home modifications are required for patients having a joint arthroplasty.

Local

Elevation in a Bradford sling (Fig. 19.1) or on a Braun's frame is very important to reduce swelling.

Distal neurovascular observations are performed to check the perfusion and function of the limb distal to the operation.

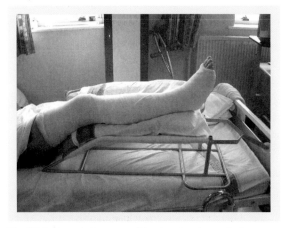

Fig. 19.1 Braun's frame used to elevate a lower limb.

Complications

General
Respiratory
Chest infections

Complications affecting the respiratory system are very common postoperatively.

A chest infection typically presents early with fever and shortness of breath. Elderly patients may be confused.

There may be signs of consolidation on examination and a low P_{O_2}.

Treatment is with physiotherapy, nebulizers and antibiotics.

Pulmonary embolus

This is the other very important chest complication.

Immobile orthopaedic patients with traumatized limbs are very susceptible to deep vein thrombosis. A variety of agents can reduce the risk including mechanical (foot pumps, graduated compression stockings) and chemical agents (heparin, clexane, aspirin, warfarin).

If the clot propagates and then breaks off it travels to the lungs (a pulmonary embolus), which can be fatal. The patient becomes acutely short of breath and has pleuritic chest pain with signs of tachycardia, tachypnoea and a low P_{O_2}.

Diagnosis is proven with a $\dot{V}/\dot{Q}$ (ventilation–perfusion) scan but treatment should not be delayed if suspected.

Intravenous anticoagulation is usually performed.

Cardiac
Myocardial infarction (MI)

MI is a relatively common postoperative complication, particularly in the elderly or those with pre-existing heart disease. The cardiac event may be silent or occur during anaesthesia and should be suspected in any patient with unexplained low blood pressure. Typically the patient will have chest pain radiating into the left arm/shoulder and be nauseous.

Diagnosis is made based on serial cardiac enzymes and electrocardiograms (ECGs).

Treatment includes oxygen and aspirin. Further agents may be used based on an opinion from the physicians (it is usually impossible to give thrombolytic drugs to postoperative patients owing to the risk of bleeding).

Left ventricular failure

This can result from a cardiac event or from aggressive fluid management over the perioperative period. It is important not to give too much fluid, particularly to elderly patients with little 'reserve'.

These patients present with shortness of breath, and signs include a raised jugular venous pressure (JVP) and bibasal crackles. Simple measures such as sitting the patient up and giving oxygen can dramatically improve the patient's condition. Further treatment includes diuretics. A medical opinion may be sought for continued management.

Gastrointestinal
Bleeding

The most important complication of the gastrointestinal (GI) system is bleeding, and the most common reason for this on the orthopaedic wards is non-steroidal anti-inflammatory drug (NSAID) therapy.

Patients with haematemesis or melaena have a suspected upper GI bleed until proven otherwise. Diagnosis is confirmed with upper GI endoscopies performed as soon as possible. Supportive measures including cross-matching of blood, fluid resuscitation, careful observations and oxygen are required.

Referral to a gastroenterologist or surgeon is needed.

Paralytic ileus

This is a less serious complication presenting with abdominal distension and nausea. Operations or trauma to the spine predispose to ileus, which usually spontaneously corrects after a few days on intravenous fluids and a nasogastric tube.

Renal
Renal failure

Pre-existing renal impairment is common in orthopaedic patients and the additional insult of a fracture or surgery with the associated blood loss can tip the balance, causing renal failure.

Factors influencing the development of renal failure include drugs (cefuroxime, diuretics, NSAIDs) and hypovolaemia. It is very important to keep patients well hydrated with enough fluid to prevent prerenal failure.

Careful monitoring of fluid input with hourly urine output and daily urea and electrolyte measurement are important when assessing such a patient.

As a junior doctor you will frequently be asked to review patients with a low urinary output postoperatively.
It is very important to carefully assess fluid balance, so that diuretics are not given to such patients just to increase the output. This may precipitate renal failure!

A patient with established renal failure needs referral to a specialist centre.

Urinary tract infection

Urinary tract infections postoperatively are very common. Diagnosis is made on urinalysis and a midstream urine (MSU) sample is sent to microbiology. Antibiotics are started until culture and sensitivity results are known.

Local

Figure 19.2 lists local complications, their timing, causes, signs and symptoms, and management.

Shock

Shock is defined as an inability to maintain adequate tissue perfusion and oxygenation.

Every doctor should be able to recognize shock.

On the orthopaedic wards the most likely causes are hypovolaemic, septic and cardiogenic shock, although neurogenic shock can occur after spinal cord injury.

Hypovolaemic

Haemorrhage is the most likely cause of hypovolaemic shock, which is due to inadequate circulatory volume.

Cardiogenic

The heart is unable to maintain adequate cardiac output, usually because of infarction.

Neurogenic/spinal

This is due to peripheral vasodilatation secondary to spinal cord injury.

Local complications of orthopaedic surgery				
Complication	Postoperative timing	Cause	Signs and symptoms	Management
Tight cast	Immediate	Swelling, dressing and/or cast too tight	Pain, tingling in toes/fingers Poor distal perfusion, numbness A tight cast can cause an ischaemic limb	Split cast and dressing Elevate limb
Compartment syndrome (see Ch. 15)	Immediate/early usually post-fracture	Swelling in closed fascial compartment	Pain, paraesthesia, pain on passive stretch, tight compartment	Pressure Measurement Fasciotomy
Infection (see Ch. 16)	Early/late	Infection at time of surgery or haematogenous seeding	Early: wound redness, discharge breakdown with ↑temperature Late: persistent pain, loosening	Early: debridement and washout Late: removal of prosthesis and debridement possible second stage reimplantation at a later stage
Dislocation of total hip replacement	Early, late	Patient: poor position, inappropriate activity Surgeon: poor stem or cup position Late: excessive wear	Severe pain Internally rotated leg (if posterior)	Reduce hip If persistent consider revision
Periprosthetic fracture	Early/late	Early: surgical complication of insertion Late: loosening of . prosthesis, infection	↑Pain, unable to bear weight	Early: fixation of fracture Late: revision of prosthesis
Nerve injury	Immediate/early	Usually retractor, e.g. sciatic nerve in hip replacement	Pain, weakness, paraesthesia	Usually await events and recovery occurs
Heterotopic ossification	Late	Bone formation in soft tissues More common in head-injured patients, hip replacement	Stiffness	NSAIDs or radiotherapy at time of surgery

Fig. 19.2 Local complications of orthopaedic surgery.

It is important not to overload such a patient with fluid in an attempt to raise the blood pressure (the BP remains low because of loss of peripheral resistance).

Septic

Peripheral vasodilatation is due to bacterial endotoxins in severe infection.

Treatment

Whatever the cause, basic treatment should be instituted immediately and includes oxygen therapy and fluid resuscitation, with catheterization to monitor urine output and regular observation.

The patient should be considered for an HDU, and further treatment is dependent on cause and severity.

- List ways of preventing complications in orthopaedic patients?
- How can you minimize infection in orthopaedic surgery?
- What is the purpose of preoperative assessment?
- Think of examples of conditions that might be discovered and be important to treat before elective orthopaedic surgery?
- How do you describe complications?
- Why is it important to examine the limb prior to surgery?
- Outline basic postoperative care.
- What must happen to any limb post-surgery?
- List as many local and general complications as you can think of?
- What is your plan for a patient with a low urinary output postoperatively?
- Define shock.
- What causes of shock are there?
- How do you treat shock?

Further reading

Fitzgerald R H, Kaufer H, Malkani A (eds) 2002 Orthopaedics. Mosby, Philadelphia

Miller M D 2000 Review of orthopaedics, 3rd edn. WB Saunders, Philadelphia

Sweetland H, Conway K 2004 Crash course in surgery. Mosby, Edinburgh

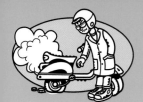
This chapter concerns bone tumours (primary and secondary) and other malignant conditions presenting as a musculoskeletal disorder.

You will notice that we have listed secondary bone tumours before primary. This is because metastatic disease of bone is far more common than primary malignancy.

- Secondary bone tumours—metastasis from:
  —Lung
  —Breast
  —Prostate
  —Kidney
  —Thyroid
  —Bowel
- Primary bone tumours:
  —Osteosarcoma
  —Ewing's sarcoma
  —Chondrosarcoma
- Soft tissue sarcomas.
- Haemopoietic diseases:
  —Myeloma
  —Leukaemia
  —Lymphoma

Secondary bone tumours

Incidence
Secondary bone tumours are the most common bone-destroying lesions in the older patient.

Aetiology and pathology
The tumours most likely to metastasize to bone are listed above. Metastatic lesions are most commonly found in the spine, pelvis, ribs and proximal long bones.

The mechanism of metastasis is shown in Figure 20.1.

Bone is destroyed by metastatic disease and weakened predisposing to fracture. The majority of metastases appear osteolytic but those from prostate cancer appear sclerotic.

Clinical features
Patient with a known primary
The patient has a clear history of previous malignancy, which in the case of breast carcinoma may have been many years previously. Unrelenting

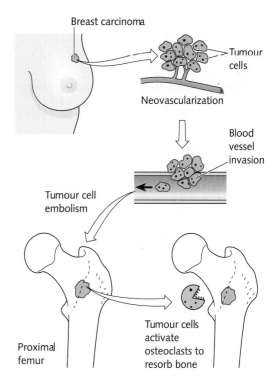

Fig. 20.1 Mechanism of long bone metastasis.

bone pain in the axial skeleton then makes the patient seek medical help. Night pain is often a feature that does not respond to simple analgesia. There may be constitutional symptoms such as weight loss and malaise.

Patient with no known primary
The patient presents with bone pain as described above but with no history of previous malignancy. In this case it is important to ask about symptoms suggestive of malignancy such as cough and haemoptysis (lung), urinary symptoms (prostate) or change in bowel habit (bowel). Patients often do not have any symptoms of the primary. Clinical examination should concentrate on likely sources of primary tumours; therefore examine:

- Breast.
- Chest.
- Prostate (per rectum).

139

- Thyroid.
- Abdomen (kidney and bowel).

Fracture
Usually the patient has a history of bone pain preceding the event (usually minor trauma) that caused the fracture. The patient is then either admitted or seen in a fracture clinic.

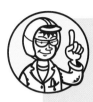 Patients who present with significant fractures after a very minor injury (e.g. after lifting a suitcase) may have a malignancy.

Spinal cord compression
Again, either of the patients above can present with weakness of the legs. Often there is a history of preceding spinal bony pain and then weakness, numbness and loss of bladder and bowel control.

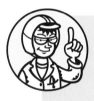 Spinal bony pain in patients with known metastatic disease needs investigation and treatment before spinal cord compression results.

Diagnosis and investigation
Any bone-destroying lesion could be due to infection or malignancy. Therefore:
- Check the white cell count (WCC) and inflammatory markers—C-reactive protein (CRP) and erythrocyte sedimentation rate (ESR). These are raised in infection but may also be raised in malignancy (myeloma).
- Further blood tests may identify the primary such as carcinoembryonic antigen (CEA) or prostate-specific antigen (PSA).
- Plain X-rays will usually show an osteolytic lesion; however, significant bone loss (>50%) is needed before it is apparent on X-ray examination.
- If strong clinical suspicion exists then an MRI scan is more sensitive.
- Cortical thinning suggests impending fracture.
- A bone scan will be hot and is useful to exclude further lesions.
- In an unknown primary, further investigation to find the primary is warranted (see Algorithm for the investigation of sinister back pain, p. 8).

Treatment
Treatment depends on the primary and on the life expectancy of the patient. A multidisciplinary approach is required involving oncologists.

Conservative
- Adequate analgesia and splintage.
- Radiotherapy is used frequently for bony metastatic pain.
- Chemotherapy may have a role in certain tumours.
- Hormonal therapy is useful in breast disease.
- Intravenous bisphosphonates are now being used to inhibit osteoclastic resorption of bone.

Surgical
- Intramedullary fixation of long bones is performed for fracture or impending fracture.
- Joint arthroplasty is sometimes used around the hip and shoulder.
- Spinal decompression and stabilization for acute cord compression.

Prognosis
The prognosis depends on the primary.

 Patients with renal tumours and a solitary metastasis may be cured by resection of both.

Primary bone tumours

Primary tumours of bone can be benign or malignant.

Benign bone tumours
Enchondroma
An enchondroma is a benign bone lesion of cartilaginous origin.

Incidence
They are quite common, occurring usually in adulthood.

Aetiology and pathology
Enchondromas develop from aberrant cartilage ('chondroma') left within bone ('en'). They are usually found in the metaphysis of long bones (femur or humerus) but are also common in the hand. See Figure 20.2.

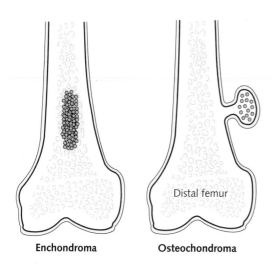

Distal femur

Enchondroma   Osteochondroma

Fig. 20.2 Benign cartilage tumours.

Clinical features
An enchondroma is usually asymptomatic and may be found incidentally. Large lesions causing cortical erosion can be painful and the patient may notice a swelling, particularly in the hand.

Diagnosis and investigation
Typical features on X-ray show a well-demarcated calcifying lesion in the metaphysis of the bone. Serial X-rays may be obtained to make sure the lesion is not growing rapidly.

Treatment
Usually no treatment is required, but if the lesion is significantly painful or associated with fracture, excision or curettage may be performed.

Osteochondroma
Incidence
This is the most common benign bone lesion, presenting from childhood through to adult life.

Aetiology and pathology
The lesion develops from aberrant cartilage remaining on the surface of the cortex. It is usually found around the knee, most commonly on the distal femur.

The pathological appearance is of a bone lesion continuous with the cortex of the bone, capped with hyaline cartilage. It can be sessile or pedunculated.

Clinical features
The majority are asymptomatic, presenting incidentally or as a swelling. Rarely, pain or pressure effects on nerves or vessels occur.

Diagnosis and investigation
The typical appearance of a pedunculated lesion in continuity with the cortex clinches the diagnosis. If there is doubt, computed tomography (CT) or magnetic resonance imaging (MRI) may reassure.

Treatment
Usually no treatment is needed; rarely, excision is carried out, if symptomatic.

Prognosis
It is extremely rare for either osteochondroma or enchondroma to undergo malignant change.

Osteoid osteoma
Osteoid osteoma is a painful self-limiting benign bone lesion.

Incidence
The lesion is uncommon, usually presenting between 5–30 years of age.

Aetiology and pathology
It is caused by a nidus of osteoblasts located in the cortex of bone, and is usually found in the tibia, spine or femur.

Clinical features
Patients have intense pain, particularly at night. Tenderness over the lesion is usual. In the spine a scoliosis may be present.

Diagnosis and investigation
X-ray features show a radiolucent nidus surrounded by a dense area of reactive bone.

CT scans confirm and accurately locate the lesion (Fig. 20.3).

Treatment
Pain relief is with non-steroidal anti-inflammatory drugs (NSAIDs).

CT-guided ablation is now preferred over surgical excision.

Prognosis
The tumour is eventually self-limiting.

Fibrous dysplasia
This is not strictly speaking a bone tumour.

Incidence
Fibrous dysplasia is relatively common, usually presenting in the first three decades.

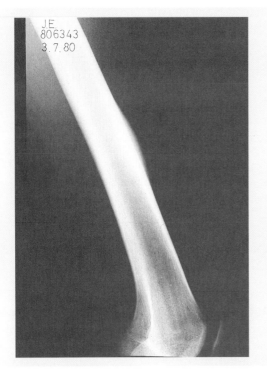

Fig. 20.3 CT scan showing an osteoid osteoma (from Hochberg M C, Silman A J, Smolen J S et al 2003 Rheumatology, 3rd edn. Mosby, Edinburgh).

Aetiology and pathology

It is most commonly found in the tibia, femur and ribs, and is caused by developmental abnormality of bone with numerous fibrous proliferations.

Clinical features

The condition is usually asymptomatic, discovered as an incidental finding, but can present with pain, swelling, deformity or fracture.

Diagnosis and investigation

A typical ground glass appearance is diagnostic.

Treatment

No treatment is usually required, but if significant, curettage and bone grafting can be performed.

Malignant primary bone tumours

Primary malignant bone tumours are very rare indeed. We will discuss two of those most likely to be encountered.

Osteosarcoma
Incidence

There are approximately 1–2 cases per million of population. Presentation is in adolescence and young

adulthood or in the elderly where they develop in Pagetic bones.

Aetiology and pathology

Paget's disease or radiation can predispose, but most cases occur sporadically. The tumour is highly malignant and secretes osteoid. Local spread occurs quickly, destroying the cortex, but it may also metastasize.

The most common location is around the knee; other sites include the proximal humerus and femur.

Clinical features

The patient presents with pain and sometimes also swelling. Clinically there is usually warmth over the affected area and there may be a palpable mass.

Diagnosis and investigation

X-rays (Fig. 20.4) may show:
- An ill-defined lesion with an indistinct zone of transition.
- Sclerotic or lytic areas within the lesion.
- Cortical destruction.
- Codman's triangle (elevation of periosteum).
- 'Sunray spicules' (calcification within the tumour but out of the bone).

Biopsy may be necessary to confirm the diagnosis. Further investigations such as CT and MRI are required to stage the lesion.

Treatment

A combined multidisciplinary team approach is adopted.

Preoperative chemotherapy followed by limb salvage surgery is performed if possible. Occasionally amputation is required.

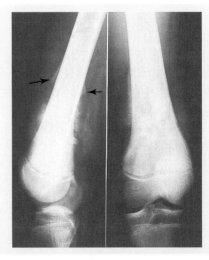

Fig. 20.4 X-ray of osteosarcoma (from Klippel J H, Dieppe P A (eds) 1998 Rheumatology, 2nd edn. Mosby, London).

Prognosis
5-year survival is 60%.

Ewing's sarcoma
Incidence
Ewing's sarcoma is extremely rare (less common than osteosarcoma), occurring between 5–25 years of age.

Aetiology and pathology
Histologically this is a small cell sarcoma. It occurs as frequently in flat bones as in long bones, being most common in the femur or tibia (long bone), pelvis or vertebra (flat bones).

These tumours are highly malignant and often large at presentation.

Clinical features
Patients present with pain and may be unwell with a fever. Clinically the area is warm and swelling may be present.

Diagnosis and investigation
Diagnosis is usually made on X-ray appearance (Fig. 20.5), which is classically a lytic lesion with a laminated periosteal reaction (onion skinning).

CT and MRI help to stage the lesion.

Biopsy may be necessary.

Treatment
A combined multidisciplinary team approach is adopted.

Preoperative chemotherapy and radiotherapy followed by limb salvage surgery is performed if possible.

Prognosis
5-year survival is 60%.

Haemopoietic diseases

Lymphoma and myeloma can present with bone destruction.

Lymphoma
Incidence
Lymphoma is rare but can occur at any age.

Aetiology and pathology
It is a small cell bone tumour arising from the marrow, which can occur in any bone, most commonly around the knee.

Diagnosis and investigation
- X-rays show a long lesion with mottled bony destruction.
- Isotope bone scanning excludes further lesions.
- Biopsy confirms the diagnosis.

Treatment
Chemotherapy and irradiation are commonly used in conjunction.

Myeloma
Incidence
This is a rare tumour occurring between 50–80 years of age.

Aetiology and pathology
Lesions are due to a plasma cell malignancy, and are found usually in the spine, ribs or clavicle.

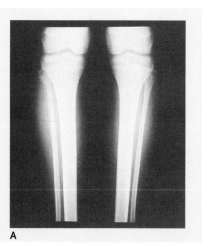
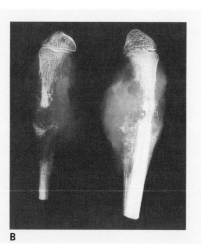

Fig. 20.5 X-ray of Ewing's sarcoma (from Hochberg M C, Silman A J, Smolen J S et al 2003 Rheumatology, 3rd edn. Mosby, Edinburgh).

A   B

Clinical features

Bony pain is common and there may be a pathological fracture. Systemic symptoms of fatigue and fever are very common.

Diagnosis and investigation

Patients will have a high erythrocyte sedimentation rate (ESR) and may have hypercalcaemia. Serum electrophoresis and urinary analysis for Bence Jones proteins confirm the diagnosis.

X-rays show classic punched-out lytic lesions.

Treatment

Chemotherapy is the mainstay with surgical stabilization or radiotherapy for impending fracture.

Prognosis

Overall prognosis is poor, with survival averaging 2 years.

Leukaemia

The last malignancy to mention is leukaemia—a malignancy of white blood cells.

Leukaemia is the most common malignancy of childhood and about one-third of patients have bone pain. Leukaemia can also present with an acutely hot, swollen joint very similar to septic arthritis.

- Which tumours most commonly metastasize to bone and why?
- How do tumour cells enter the circulation?
- With what symptoms can patients with metastatic bone disease present?
- What investigations are useful to confirm the presence of bony secondaries?
- What features on X-ray are typical of a secondary deposit?
- What treatment is available for secondary malignancy?
- Are any patients with a secondary lesion still curable?
- List all the causes of abnormal bone you can think of?
- Name as many benign bone tumours as you can?
- What is the difference between an enchondroma and an osteochondroma?
- How does an osteoid osteoma present and how do you treat it?
- What is the classical X-ray appearance of fibrous dysplasia?
- Name two malignant bone tumours?
- Explain the different X-ray features between benign and malignant tumours?
- How do you treat malignant bone tumours and what is the survival?
- Name some other malignant conditions that can affect the musculoskeletal system?

Further reading

Dandy D J 1998 Essentials of orthopaedics and trauma, 3rd edn. Churchill Livingstone, London
Fitzgerald R H, Kaufer H, Malkani A (eds) 2002 Orthopaedics. Mosby, Philadelphia
Miller M D 2000 Review of orthopaedics, 3rd edn. WB Saunders, Philadelphia

Solomon L, Warwick D, Nayagan D (eds) 2001 Apley's system of orthopaedics and fractures, 8th edn. Hodder Arnold, London
Orthoteers website: http://www.orthoteers.co.uk

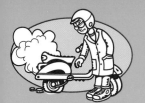

Musculoskeletal back pain

Back pain is extremely common and causes a significant burden on the resources of westernized societies in terms of lost working days.

Definition
Musculoskeletal back pain is not a single specific disease entity but rather a collection of ill-defined conditions presenting with low back pain. This diagnosis should only be made after other pathological conditions have been excluded.

Incidence
60–80% of the population will have back pain at some stage in their lives.

Aetiology and pathology
As back pain is so common it is difficult to define clear aetiological factors for its occurrence.

It is known, however, that patients with chronic back pain are more likely to smoke, have a medico-legal claim pending and be over 30 at presentation.

There is much controversy about the exact pathology involved in back pain. One of the problems is that a lot of the pathological changes seen will also be present in the healthy 'normal' population with no symptoms.

Implicated structures are listed in Figure 21.1.
- Facet joint arthritis shows the typical features of osteoarthritis (OA) with joint space destruction and osteophyte formation.
- Degenerative disc disease occurs with ageing and is related to decreased water content in the nucleus pulposus. The disc space narrows and the segment is said to become more mobile. It is this abnormal movement, together with an inability to distribute load, that causes pain.

Possible causes of musculoskeletal back pain

Bone/periosteum
Paraspinous muscles spasm/sprain
Facet joint arthritis
Disc/degenerative disc disease
Posterior longitudinal ligament

Fig. 21.1 Possible causes of musculoskeletal back pain.

An interesting point is that patients rarely present after the age of 60 and as the patient enters old age usually the symptoms subside. This is said to be due to stiffening of a mobile spine.

Clinical features
There are two typical clinical scenarios.

An acutely presenting patient with a history of back pain over days or weeks
Pain is usually solely located to the back, possibly following a precipitating incident.

It is a severe pain and the patient may have difficulty getting into a comfortable position. Sometimes the patient has pain referred down the back of the leg but this differs from true sciatica (radicular pain) in that back pain is still the predominant feature and the pain does not radiate to the foot.

The pain is mechanical (i.e. worse on movement).

Clinical examination will show muscle spasm with loss of lumbar lordosis. The patient may find it difficult to walk and spinal movements will be almost entirely lost.

Sciatic stretch testing and peripheral nerve examination will be negative.

The chronic patient who has unrelenting back pain for many years
The patient will be unable to work, may be overweight and depressed. Usually the patient has seen numerous doctors, physiotherapists and other allied health workers including alternative medical practitioners.

The back pain is usually unrelenting and does not have any relieving factors. Leg pain may or may not be present.

Clinical examination rarely shows any significant features other than reduced movements. Inappropriate signs (Waddell's signs) may be present (e.g. increased pain on applying mild downward pressure to the head).

Diagnosis and investigation
The majority of patients with a short history (less than 6 weeks) and mechanical symptoms need no further investigation.

Prolonged symptoms need investigation to exclude other causes of back pain listed below, including malignancy.

Blood tests including full blood count (FBC), liver function tests (LFTs), calcium, myeloma screen, erythrocyte sedimentation rate (ESR) and C-reactive protein (CRP) should all be normal in mechanical back pain.

X-rays if performed may show:
- Normal appearances.
- Minor disc narrowing.
- Facet joint arthritis (Fig. 21.2).

Magnetic resonance imaging (MRI) or computed tomography (CT) scanning are rarely helpful and may be misleading if they highlight an abnormality that may not be significant.

Treatment
Conservative
Analgesia, non-steroidal anti-inflammatory drugs (NSAIDs) and physiotherapy are used for acute low back pain. Prolonged bed rest should be avoided.

Chronic patients are very difficult to treat and need a multidisciplinary approach to try to break the pain cycle. Psychological input may be required, as may the 'pain team'. Occasionally facet joint injections for localized disease can relieve symptoms.

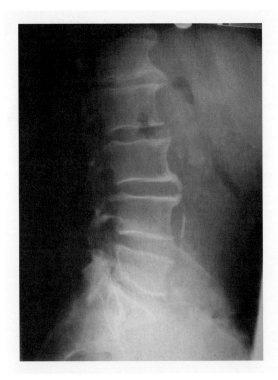

Fig. 21.2 Osteoarthritis of the spine.

Surgical
This is controversial but some advocate spinal fusion in a few very selected patients with degenerative disc disease.

Prognosis
Most acute back pain episodes settle spontaneously and the patient returns to normal.

Once chronic, the condition becomes extremely difficult to treat.

Prolapsed intervertebral disc

Definition
A disc prolapse occurs when part of the nucleus pulposus herniates through the annulus fibrosus and presses on a spinal nerve root.

Incidence
Disc prolapse is common—up to 3% of men and 1% of women will suffer with sciatica related to a prolapsed intervertebral disc. Usual presentation is between 35 and 55 years of age.

Aetiology and pathology
There is good evidence that manual workers involved in heavy lifting have increased incidence of disc prolapse. Regular automobile use is also said to be a risk factor.

The herniation of disc material tends to occur posterolaterally where the annulus is thinner. Central disc prolapse can occur and press on the combined nerve roots (including those supplying the bladder and bowel). This is called the cauda equina syndrome.

Prolapse can occur without spinal root involvement in which case the patient will have symptoms of back pain and perhaps referred pain but not true sciatica.

Disc prolapse most commonly occurs at L4–L5 or L5–S1 level but can occur at any level (including cervical and rarely thoracic). The nerve root crosses its space before exiting the spine beneath the pedicle (L4–L5 disc presses on L5 nerve root). See Figure 21.3.

Clinical features
Sciatica is a symptom of nerve root irritation. The patient complains of severe pain radiating down the leg into the toes. There may be numbness and tingling in the foot and weakness of the foot. Patients

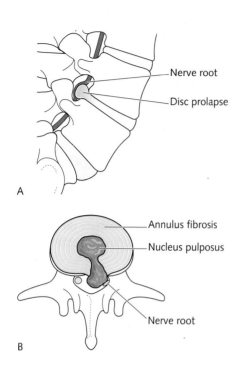

Nerve root

Disc prolapse

A

Annulus fibrosis

Nucleus pulposus

Nerve root

B

Fig. 21.3 Prolapsed intervertebral disc.

find it very uncomfortable to sit, and either stand or lie down. Coughing and sneezing worsen the pain.

In cauda equina syndrome there is bladder and bowel dysfunction with possibly urinary retention and saddle anaesthesia.

 Bilateral leg symptoms are suggestive of impending cauda equina.

Clinically a patient will have an abnormal posture, stooping to the affected side and standing with the knee flexed to relieve pressure on the dura (Fig. 21.4).

Nerve root tension signs such as straight leg raising will be positive.

The crossover sign may be positive (elevation of the opposite or normal leg gives pain shooting down the affected leg).

Numbness in a dermatomal distribution and weakness with loss of reflexes may be present.

In cauda equina there is loss of anal tone and reduced perianal sensation.

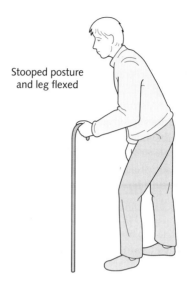

Stooped posture and leg flexed

Fig. 21.4 Posture in prolapsed intervertebral disc.

Diagnosis and investigation

In older patients blood tests described above should be performed to exclude any sinister causes.

X-rays are usually normal and are performed to exclude bony pathology such as spondylolisthesis.

MRI scanning is now the investigation of choice in patients with persistent symptoms (Fig. 21.5).

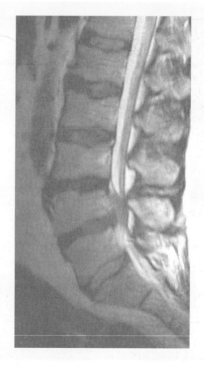

Fig. 21.5 MRI scan of prolapsed intervertebral disc at L4–L5 level.

147

Surgical

Severe symptoms not responding to conservative measures require surgical decompression.

Prognosis

The condition tends to be progressive.

Discitis/vertebral osteomyelitis

Definition

Discitis is infection of the disc space, and vertebral osteomyelitis infection of a vertebral body. The two often go hand in hand and it is often impossible to distinguish them.

Incidence

They are becoming more common, although still rare.

Presentation can be at any age from child to elderly.

Aetiology and pathology

Conditions associated with other bone and joint infection (see Ch. 16), particularly intravenous drug use and immunocompromised patients, predispose to spinal infection. Any patient with a recent septicaemic episode from pneumonia or urinary tract infection (UTI) can subsequently develop discitis by seeding of infection.

Common infecting organisms are *Staphylococcus aureus* and streptococci but tuberculosis should be considered.

Clinical features

Patients are unwell with a pyrexia and complain of severe unrelenting back pain. They may have another chronic debilitating disease such as renal failure.

Clinical examination may reveal a swelling over the affected area and in severe cases a gibbus (kyphotic deformity resulting from vertebral collapse) may be present. Pain on palpation will be present and movements lost.

One of the common features of discitis is that it presents late, often the patient having 6–12 weeks of symptoms before the correct diagnosis is made. Abnormal neurology may be present.

Diagnosis and investigation

The white cell count (WCC) is elevated as are the ESR and CRP.

X-rays show narrowed disc space and bony destruction (Fig. 21.9).

An isotope bone scan will be hot in the affected area and is a good screening test in a patient with an infection.

MRI scanning should be performed to detect any epidural abscess.

Biopsy should be obtained for culture and sensitivity (can be done under X-ray or CT guidance).

Treatment
Conservative

Intravenous antibiotics are given for 6 weeks.

Surgical

Any abscess should be drained and an unstable spine with significant deformity needs stabilization.

Prognosis

Prognosis is variable: childhood cases respond well and should return to normality; severe adult infections can be life-threatening and surgery carries significant risk.

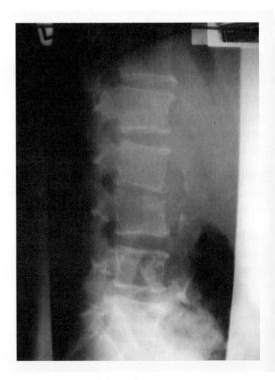

Fig. 21.9 Discitis with bony destruction.

Scoliosis

Definition
This is a lateral deviation and rotational abnormality of the spine.

Incidence
Up to 2.5% of the population are affected by idiopathic scoliosis.

Aetiology and pathology
Causes of scoliosis are listed in Figure 21.10.

In idiopathic scoliosis the exact cause is not known.

Curves are thoracolumbar (Fig. 21.11).

Clinical features
Pain is not usually a feature; rather the patient or relatives complain of deformity, in the form of an asymmetrical rib hump, spinal curve and limb length inequality. For clinical examination, the rib hump is more prominent on forward flexion (Fig. 21.12).

Very severe deformity reduces chest expansion which can be life-threatening.

Diagnosis and investigation
X-rays (standing posteroanterior (PA) and lateral) show the curve, and serial films are important to monitor the progress of the curve.

A significant increase in the severity of the curve is often an indication for surgical stabilization.

MRI scans are performed to exclude any associated spinal cord abnormality.

Treatment
Conservative
The treatment depends on the angle of the curve measured on the X-rays. In idiopathic scoliosis the

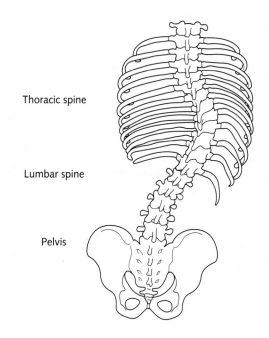

Thoracic spine

Lumbar spine

Pelvis

Fig. 21.11 Thoracolumbar curve in scoliosis.

initial treatment is bracing for mild to moderate curves.

Surgical
All congenital, most neuromuscular and severe or progressive idiopathic curves will require surgical stabilization, fusion and correction.

Correction of deformity carries a real risk of complete paraplegia.

Prognosis
The majority of curves are minor and require little treatment.

Very severe neuromuscular curves can lead to death due to cardiorespiratory compromise.

Fig. 21.10 Causes of scoliosis.

Causes of scoliosis		
Type	**Pathology**	**Example**
Congenital	Abnormal development of spine	Hemivertebra
Idiopathic	Unknown	Adolescent idiopathic scoliosis
Neuromuscular	Abnormal muscle forces acting on the spine	Cerebral palsy
Secondary	Curve develops secondary to another process	Leg length discrepancy

Fig. 21.12 Examination of a patient with scoliosis.

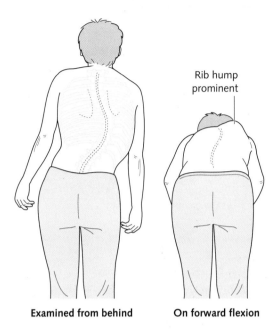

Rib hump
prominent

Examined from behind   On forward flexion

- Discuss the likely causes of back pain.
- What features of back pain would make you think of a sinister cause?
- Discuss the causes, presentation and treatment of musculoskeletal back pain.
- Why do we investigate back pain? When? And how?
- What features in the history suggest prolapsed intervertebral disc?
- How does spinal stenosis differ from prolapsed intervertebral disc?
- What is the pathology in a disc prolapse?
- Where is the nerve root compressed?
- What is the likely outcome?
- What other condition can be confused with spinal stenosis and how can you exclude it with investigations?
- How does discitis present?
- Who is more at risk of discitis?
- How do you investigate and treat discitis?
- When is surgery required?
- What different types of scoliosis are there?
- What features do you look for clinically?
- What do you use to guide treatment?
- What is the main risk of surgery?

Further reading

Dandy D J 1998 Essentials of orthopaedics and trauma, 3rd edn. Churchill Livingstone, London

Fitzgerald R H, Kaufer H, Malkani A (eds) 2002 Orthopaedics. Mosby, Philadelphia

Miller M D 2000 Review of orthopaedics, 3rd edn. WB Saunders, Philadelphia

Solomon L, Warwick D, Nayagan D (eds) 2001 Apley's system of orthopaedics and fractures, 8th edn. Hodder Arnold, London

Orthoteers website: http://www.orthoteers.co.uk

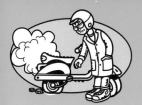

22. Sports Injuries

Knee injuries

Introduction
The knee is commonly injured in sport—particularly football (soccer), rugby and skiing.

In the first part of this chapter we will discuss injuries to the menisci, ligamentous injuries of the knee and patellar dislocation.

Meniscal injuries
The menisci are two semicircular fibrocartilage structures that lie between the femoral and tibial articular surfaces (Fig. 22.1). Essentially they act as 'shock absorbers' and are prone to injuries due to the large forces crossing the knee.

Incidence
Meniscal injuries are common, usually occurring in young adult patients who participate in sports.

Pathology and aetiology
The medial meniscus is more commonly injured because the lateral meniscus is more mobile.

A discoid lateral meniscus is abnormally large and more likely to tear.

Meniscal tears can be traumatic or degenerative:

- Traumatic tears. The meniscus is normal and injury usually occurs after landing or twisting with the knee flexed. The injury can be associated with a ligamentous injury such as anterior cruciate ligament (ACL) tear (usually the lateral meniscus). A chronically unstable knee is prone to further tears.
- Degenerative tears. These occur in an older population through abnormal cartilage. They may occur with little or no injury.

Types of meniscal tears (Fig. 22.2)
1. Bucket handle. The tear extends over a distance, remaining attached at the anterior and posterior horns. It can be displaced (in which case the cartilage flips over) or undisplaced (the cartilage remains in its normal position). A locked knee results when a large bucket handle tear flips over and becomes trapped in the joint, resulting in loss of complete extension.
2. Radial.
3. Horizontal cleavage.
4. Flap/parrot beak.

Of clinical importance is how peripheral the tear is. Very peripheral tears occur through vascular tissue and are amenable to repair, as these tears can heal.

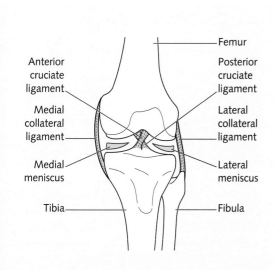

Fig. 22.1 Basic anatomy of the knee.

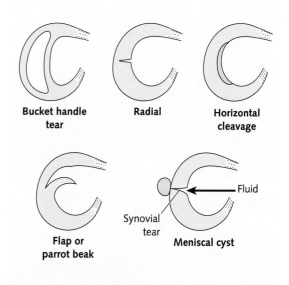

Fig. 22.2 Meniscal lesions.

Meniscal tears further away from the blood supply (i.e. further into the knee) cannot heal.

Meniscal cysts result from synovial fluid being pumped into the meniscal tear. A valve effect means the fluid in the cyst cannot drain back into the knee. See Fig. 22.2.

Clinical features

Patients usually give a history of injury while playing sport, the incident occurring during a tackle or when twisting or changing direction.

There is a range of patient presentations. A patient may present immediately after injury with a painful locked knee, or with a gradual chronic nagging pain over months or years following minor injury. This variation reflects how the different types and positions of tears manifest clinical symptoms.

Mechanical symptoms such as locking and catching suggest meniscal pathology. A 'clicking joint' does not necessarily mean there is pathology.

A more major injury with acute swelling and instability suggests associated ligamentous injury.

Examination may reveal:

- A locked knee.
- An effusion:
  —a large acute effusion suggests a very peripheral tear (which bleeds) or an associated injury
  —a small chronic effusion is common.
- Joint line tenderness; this is an important part of the examination and is usually positive in a patient with a torn meniscus.
- A meniscal cyst, which may be palpable over the lateral joint line.

A variety of special tests are described for meniscal tears and none is very reliable.

Diagnosis and investigation

In most cases the diagnosis is made solely on the basis of history and examination.

X-rays are usually normal and are performed to exclude osteoarthritis or other rare causes of knee pain.

Magnetic resonance imaging (MRI) is very useful to confirm the presence of torn menisci, particularly in patients with a dubious history.

The most accurate way to confirm the diagnosis is with arthroscopy of the knee.

Management
Conservative
Initially RICE (rest, ice, compression, elevation) is used for an acutely swollen knee. Early physiotherapy is essential to encourage movement.

Surgical
Surgery is now performed using arthroscopic techniques.

For peripheral bucket handle tears, meniscal repair has the advantage of retaining the meniscus.

For tears not amenable to repair, meniscal resection is commonly performed. Partial meniscectomy removes the damaged portion only, leaving a stable rim and reducing the risk of osteoarthritis in the future.

Prognosis
Removal of the meniscus leads to osteoarthritic changes developing in the knee because of increased load on the articular surface.

Meniscal repair is successful in 70% of cases.

Ligamentous injuries of the knee
Anterior cruciate ligament (ACL)
Incidence
1 per 3000 of the population per year are affected; therefore a large district general hospital serving a population of 300 000 will see 100 cases per year.

It is more common in men overall, but women participating in sport are now thought to be more susceptible.

Aetiology and pathology
The ACL is the primary restraint to anterior tibial translation. The mechanism of injury is usually a twisting or valgus strain pattern of injury commonly occurring in soccer or skiing (Fig. 22.3).

The knee is usually extended or slightly flexed with the foot fixed. Associated injuries to the medial collateral ligament and either meniscus are common.

ACL-deficient knees are liable to further meniscal tears.

Clinical features
Patients usually present with an acutely swollen knee following a sporting injury.

Unlike with some meniscal injuries, the patient will be unable to play on and may have to be carried from the field.

The injury may occur whilst changing direction quickly and the patient often hears a 'pop' or feels 'something go' inside the knee.

Swelling typically occurs rapidly (within 1 hour).

Once initial symptoms have settled, the patient may complain of giving way of the knee. This occurs when the patient tries to turn rapidly. Classically the

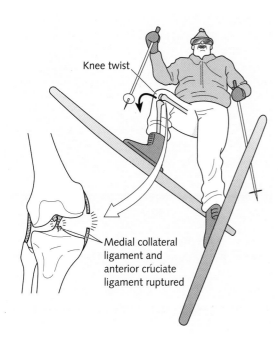

Knee twist

Medial collateral ligament and anterior cruciate ligament ruptured

Fig. 22.3 Mechanism of injury in ACL rupture.

patient will report being able to run in a straight line but not able to 'twist and turn'.

Often patients present months or years after the initial injury and may have had recurrent meniscal tears.

Clinically, patients have a tense effusion.

Range of movement is usually restricted due to pain and swelling.

The anterior drawer, Lachmann's and pivot shift tests are positive (see Ch. 27).

Diagnosis and investigation

The majority can be diagnosed clinically on the basis of history and examination.

In some patients it is difficult to elicit positive examination findings and in those patients an MRI scan or examination under anaesthetic (EUA) is useful to confirm the diagnosis.

The diagnosis is often made at arthroscopy for suspected meniscal tear.

X-rays will usually be normal.

Management
Conservative

Initial treatment is with RICE and physiotherapy. A proportion of patients can modify their activities and manage with a hamstring rehabilitation programme only.

Surgical

Any associated meniscal pathology should be addressed arthroscopically.

Operative reconstruction of the ligament is performed for functional instability.

Prognosis

Chronic instability associated with meniscal pathology leads to early osteoarthritis (OA). There is no evidence that ACL reconstruction can prevent OA developing in the future.

Posterior cruciate ligament (PCL)

The PCL is the primary restraint to posterior movement of the tibia on the femur.

Incidence

PCL injuries are rare.

Aetiology and pathology

PCL injuries occur either in sporting activities or from road traffic accidents (dashboard injury) (Fig. 22.4).

Classically it is a goalkeeper's injury in soccer, the mechanism of injury being the knee combining with an onrushing attacking player forcing the tibia backwards. The PCL can also rupture when the knee is forcibly hyperextended.

The majority of PCL tears occur in combination with other ligamentous injuries.

Clinical features

The patient will have a substantial injury to the knee and will usually be unable to bear weight. Swelling is usually less obvious than with an ACL injury.

Patients complain less of instability than with ACL injuries.

Clinically, patients will have a posterior sag and positive posterior drawer test.

Careful assessment is needed to look for associated injuries such as lateral collateral injuries.

Treatment
Conservative

Almost all isolated PCL injuries can be treated with rehabilitation alone.

Surgical

Patients with combined injuries or symptomatic instability require reconstruction.

Prognosis

In the short term PCL injuries often follow a benign course and are often asymptomatic in certain sports players (a professional rugby league team will have several players who are PCL deficient).

Osteoarthritis develops in the long term (25 years).

Fig. 22.4 Mechanism of injury in PCL injuries.

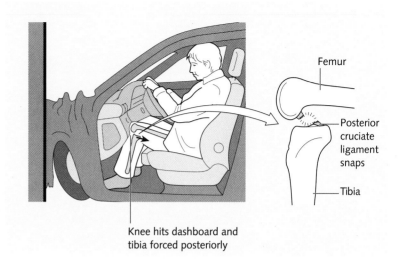

Femur

Posterior cruciate ligament snaps

Tibia

Knee hits dashboard and tibia forced posteriorly

Lateral collateral injuries
Incidence
These are rare injuries.

Aetiology and pathology
Isolated lateral collateral ligament (LCL) injuries occur when a varus strain is placed on the knee (i.e. a hit from the medial side) (Fig. 22.5).

Associated injuries to the PCL or ACL can occur.

Clinical features
The patient will complain of pain and possibly instability.

In the normal knee the LCL is easily palpable as a cord-like structure. When the LCL is ruptured, the area is tender and indistinct.

Opening up of the joint on the lateral side will be present on collateral testing.

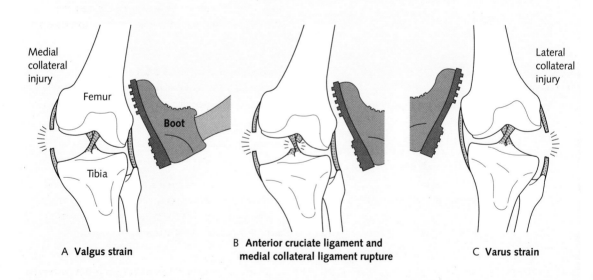

Medial collateral injury

Femur

Boot

Tibia

Lateral collateral injury

A **Valgus strain**

B **Anterior cruciate ligament and medial collateral ligament rupture**

C **Varus strain**

Fig. 22.5 Mechanism of injury in collateral ligament tears.

Management

Almost all isolated injuries heal well with conservative treatment.

Prognosis

The knee should return to normal.

Medial collateral injuries

Incidence

These are common injuries in isolation or combined with ACL injury.

Aetiology and pathology

There is a valgus strain pattern of injury. The injury can be complete or partial, and can be associated with ACL injury.

Clinical features

This is usually a sporting injury; the patient may hear 'something go' but an effusion is *not* a feature of an isolated medial collateral ligament (MCL) tear (it is an extra-articular structure).

Tenderness over the broad attachment of the MCL and opening up of the joint on collateral stressing are examination features.

Management

Treatment is with physiotherapy, with bracing initially if required. The injury usually heals well with conservative treatment.

Surgical advancement is sometimes required for chronic unstable injuries.

Prognosis

The knee usually returns to normal after a period of rehabilitation.

Patellar dislocation

Introduction

The patella is prevented from dislocation by anatomical features such as a large lateral femoral condyle and the insertion of vastus medialis oblique (VMO) (Fig. 22.6).

Incidence

Patellar dislocation is quite common.

Aetiology and pathology

Patellar dislocation can be habitual or traumatic.

Habitual dislocators are often young women with ligamentous laxity and a hypoplastic femoral condyle. This group get recurrent dislocations after minor injuries and are difficult to treat.

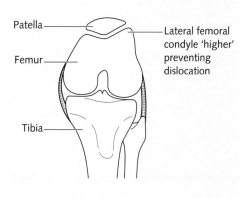

Fig. 22.6 Anatomical features that prevent lateral dislocation of the patella.

Traumatic dislocations occur during sports, usually with the knee slightly flexed with side impact. The dislocation occurs laterally and damage may occur to the joint surface. Structures along the medial border of the patella are torn.

Clinical features

A first-time dislocation is extremely painful and the patient arrives in casualty with the patella laterally placed.

Often there is tenderness over the medial side of the knee and an effusion.

Later when the acute injury has settled the patient may have patella apprehension and a J-sign (see Ch. 27).

Diagnosis and investigation

X-rays should be taken after reduction, including a tunnel and skyline view looking for any osteochondral defects.

Management

Conservative

Initial reduction is required, usually under sedation in the accident and emergency (A&E) department.

Following this, a short period of immobilization and physiotherapy is required.

Surgical

Large osteochondral defects should be repaired or removed arthroscopically.

Recurrent dislocations may require surgical realignment.

Shoulder dislocation

Incidence
The shoulder is the most commonly dislocated large joint in the body.

Aetiology and pathology
The shoulder is at risk of dislocation because the joint has very little inherent bony stability, with reliance instead on capsule, ligaments and rotator cuff muscles. The joint has 'sacrificed' stability for movement.

The dislocation can be anterior or posterior. Anterior dislocation (Fig. 22.7) accounts for 98% and usually occurs when the arm is forced back in a position of external rotation and abduction.

Posterior dislocations occur in epileptics and electrocutions.

In anterior dislocation the capsule is damaged antero-inferiorly, leaving a so-called Bankart lesion predisposing to further dislocations. Recurrent dislocations cause a Hill–Sachs lesion due to impaction of the glenoid on the posterior part of the humeral head.

In older patients the rotator cuff is torn rather than a Bankart lesion developing.

Clinical features
The patient is often a sports player—typically rugby—and has an acute injury to the shoulder as

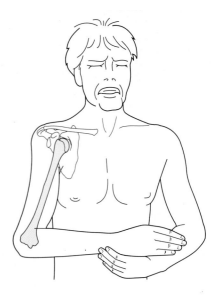

Fig. 22.8 Abnormal shoulder contour in anterior dislocation of the humerus.

described above. The injury is intensely painful and the shoulder is held supported by the other arm (Fig. 22.8). Patients will often know they have dislocated their shoulder, as opposed to another form of injury.

Examination findings include:
- Loss of normal contour.
- Palpable glenoid.
- Complete loss of movement.

Diagnosis and investigation
Anterior dislocation is usually obvious and confirmed with X-rays (also performed to exclude a fracture).

Posterior dislocation is often missed as the initial anteroposterior (AP) X-ray looks normal to the untrained eye.

The 'light bulb sign' (Fig. 22.9A) should raise suspicion but the diagnosis is made on axillary view (Fig. 22.9B) or CT scan.

Treatment
Conservative
The dislocation needs to be promptly reduced in the A&E department under sedation. A variety of methods are described.

Posterior dislocation needs a general anaesthetic and may need open reduction.

Once the dislocation is reduced, the joint is immobilized for a short period prior to supervised early rehabilitation with the physiotherapist.

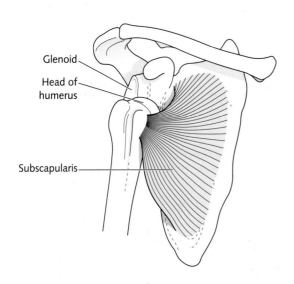

Glenoid

Head of humerus

Subscapularis

Fig. 22.7 Anterior dislocation of the humerus.

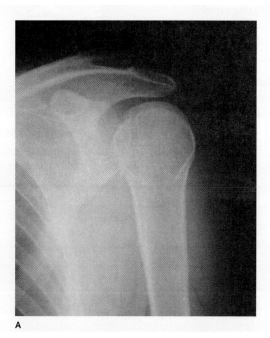

A

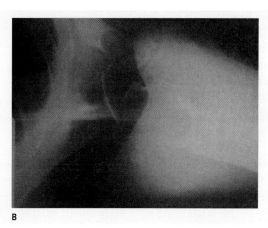

B

Fig. 22.9 Posterior dislocation of the shoulder: (A) AP X-ray showing the 'light bulb' sign; (B) axillary view.

 Your current textbook may advise 6 weeks' immobilization for patellar and shoulder dislocations to allow the 'soft tissues to heal'. This is old-fashioned thinking and a short period of rest (3–5 days) is now followed by early rehabilitation.

Ankle sprain

Incidence
This is a very common injury.

Aetiology and pathology
The injury is commonly found on the sports field but anyone can have an ankle sprain. The mechanism of injury is inversion with damage to the lateral ligament complex.

As the talus tilts in the ankle mortice, the anterior talofibular and calcaneofibular ligaments are torn (Fig. 22.10).

Clinical features
The patient experiences pain and may feel 'something go'; swelling occurs rapidly.

Chronic ankle instability leads to giving way of the joint.

Clinically the patient has a variable amount of swelling and tenderness over the lateral ligament complex.

Surgical
Surgery is usually reserved for the recurrent dislocator although some now advocate early arthroscopic examination, particularly in the young athlete.

Prognosis
A young male sportsman has an 80% chance of recurrent dislocation following anterior dislocation of the shoulder.

In the more elderly population shoulder stiffness is more of a problem than recurrence.

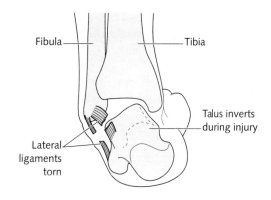

Fig. 22.10 Ankle ligament rupture.

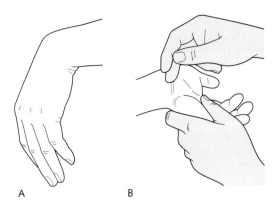

Fig. 23.3 Provocation tests for carpal tunnel syndrome may reproduce the patient's symptoms. (A) Phalen's test: the wrist is held in maximal palmar flexion. (B) Tinel's test: tap over the median nerve proximal to the transverse carpal ligament in the wrist.

Ulnar nerve entrapment

Definition
The ulnar nerve can become compressed as it passes behind the medial epicondyle or through Guyon's canal in the wrist.

Incidence
Ulnar nerve damage at the elbow is fairly common, because of its superficial position.

Aetiology
Ulnar nerve entrapment may be idiopathic or due to a precipitating cause (see Fig. 23.4).

Clinical features
Patients develop pain and/or paraesthesiae in the medial side of the elbow, which radiates to the medial forearm and the ulnar nerve distribution in the hand (see Fig. 23.2). The pain is often exacerbated by elbow flexion.

Examination usually reveals reduced sensation in the ulnar nerve distribution. Palpation of the nerve behind the medial epicondyle may provoke the symptoms. Motor dysfunction may result in atrophy

---

Precipitating factors for ulnar nerve entrapment

Local trauma, e.g. fractures of the elbow
Prolonged leaning on the elbow
Elbow synovitis

Fig. 23.4 Precipitating factors for ulnar nerve entrapment.

162

---

of the hypothenar eminence. Abduction and adduction of the fingers is weak. There may be clawing of the hand due to weakness of the intrinsic muscles (Fig. 23.5).

Investigations
Nerve conduction studies confirm the diagnosis and establish the site of compression.

Management
Ulnar nerve compression due to elbow synovitis may respond to corticosteroid injection of the elbow. Surgical decompression should be performed if sensory symptoms cannot be tolerated or if there is muscle weakness or wasting.

Radial nerve injuries

Aetiology
Radial nerve compression in the axilla is typically seen in a drunk person who falls asleep with an arm hanging over the back of a chair ('Saturday night palsy'). The radial nerve may also be injured by fractures of the humerus.

Clinical features
The wrist extensors are paralysed, resulting in wrist drop. Grip strength is dramatically reduced, as the finger flexors do not function well with the wrist in a flexed position. Nerve injury in the axilla will also lead to paralysis of the triceps. Sensory loss only affects a small area of skin on the dorsum of the hand.

Management
The wrist should be splinted immediately and the cause of the radial nerve palsy should be assessed. If

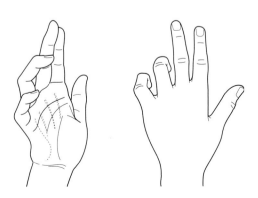

Fig. 23.5 Clawing of the hand due to ulnar nerve palsy.

there is no resolution, tendon transfer or nerve grafting may be indicated.

Common peroneal nerve injuries

Aetiology
The common peroneal nerve winds around the neck of the fibula and is in a vulnerable position. It may be damaged by fractures of the neck of fibula or pressure from a tight bandage or plaster cast.

Clinical features
Common peroneal nerve injury results in paralysis of the ankle and foot extensors. Unopposed action of the foot flexors and inverters cause the foot to be plantar flexed and inverted. This is referred to as 'foot drop'. Patients develop a high-stepping gait, flicking the foot forwards to avoid tripping over it. There is also loss of sensation over the anterior and lateral sides of the leg and the dorsum of the foot and toes.

Management
Pressure on the nerve should be relieved and a splint should be applied. If the foot drop does not resolve, an ankle–foot orthosis can be used to maintain some degree of dorsiflexion.

- List the conditions that predispose to carpal tunnel syndrome.
- What clinical signs may be found on examination of a patient with carpal tunnel syndrome?
- Understand the sensory innervation of the hand.
- Describe the gait of a patient with a common peroneal nerve injury.

Further reading
Nashel D J 2003 Entrapment neuropathies and compartment syndromes. In: Hochberg et al (eds) *Rheumatology*, 3rd edn. Mosby, London, p 713–724

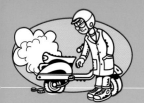

24. Soft Tissue Disorders

Introduction
Soft tissue disorders are common. They are responsible for many days of absence from work and contribute significantly to the workload in primary care, accident and emergency departments, and rheumatology and orthopaedic clinics. This chapter will discuss the presentation, diagnosis and management of some common soft tissue lesions.

Tendon lesions

The three main pathologies that affect tendons are:
- Tendinitis.
- Tenosynovitis.
- Rupture.

Tendinitis
Definition
Pain arises from strain or injury to tendons and their insertions to bone. The term 'enthesopathy' is used to describe cases with a significant periosteal component, such as lateral epicondylitis (tennis elbow).

Aetiopathogenesis
The pathogenesis of tendinitis is poorly understood. Some cases occur as part of a systemic inflammatory condition and others are related to injury from overuse. However, most cases of tendinitis are idiopathic.

Clinical features
The most frequent sites of tendinitis are the:
- Shoulder.
- Elbow.
- Achilles tendon.

Patients complain of pain that is worsened by active movement. Examination findings include:
- Tenderness of the tendon and its insertion.
- An increase in pain when active movement is performed against resistance.
- Soft tissue swelling (not always present).

An example: tennis elbow and golfer's elbow
In these conditions, pain is centred around the lateral and medial epicondyles respectively, although it may radiate distally from the elbow.

The examination findings are as follows:

Tennis elbow The origin of the forearm extensors is tender, and pain is exacerbated by resisted wrist extension (Fig. 24.1A). Pain on extension of the ring finger is particularly specific for tennis elbow.

Golfer's elbow The origin of the forearm flexors is tender, and pain is exacerbated by resisted wrist flexion (Fig. 24.1B).

Investigations of tendinitis
Tendinitis can be diagnosed clinically and investigations are often unremarkable. Radiographs may show abnormalities, such as calcification in chronic rotator cuff tendinitis. Ultrasound may also detect changes in the tendon and surrounding tissue.

Management of tendinitis
The interventions shown below may lead to improvement of symptoms. The strategies at the top of the list should be employed early in the disease process, whilst those at the bottom should be reserved for resistant cases:
- Rest or avoidance of precipitating cause.
- Non-steroidal anti-inflammatory drug (NSAID) therapy.
- Local corticosteroid injection.
- Ultrasound therapy.
- Surgery.

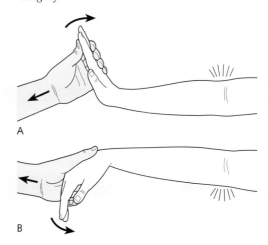

Fig. 24.1 The pain of tennis elbow is exacerbated by resisted wrist extension (A). The pain of golfer's elbow is exacerbated by resisted wrist flexion (B).

Tenosynovitis

Definition

Tenosynovitis is inflammation of the synovial lining of a tendon sheath.

Aetiology

The two main causes are:
- Inflammatory arthritis.
- Trauma.

Trauma usually results from repetitive or unaccustomed movement.

Clinical features

Patients present with pain in the region of the affected tendon. Common sites of tenosynovitis are the abductor pollicis longus and extensor pollicis brevis tendons (*De Quervain's tenosynovitis*) and finger flexors. On examination, the tendon is swollen and tender, and crepitus may be felt on palpation.

A *trigger finger* or *thumb* results from tenosynovitis of the flexor tendons. A nodule can develop on the tendon in response to constriction of the tendon sheath. The nodule 'catches' as it enters or leaves the flexor tunnel and a 'snapping' or 'flicking' movement of the digit occurs on flexion or extension.

Management

Treatment includes rest, splinting and local corticosteroid injection. Surgical decompression of the tendon sheath may be required.

Tendon rupture

Aetiology

Tendon rupture may result from chronic inflammation and degeneration or trauma. For example, rupture of the extensor tendons of the fingers is often seen in rheumatoid arthritis.

Clinical features

The resulting clinical features are loss of movement at the joint to which the tendon provides power, deformity and sometimes swelling. After rupture of the biceps tendon, a bulge formed by the lateral muscle belly is seen in the upper arm. Extensor tendon rupture at the distal end of the finger can occur when catching a cricket ball. It results in flexion of the distal interphalangeal (DIP) joint ('Mallet finger') (Fig. 24.2).

Management

Surgery can often be performed to repair the tendon and restore function.

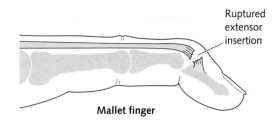

Fig. 24.2 'Mallet finger'.

Bursitis

Bursae are small sacs of fibrous tissue that are lined with synovial membrane, which secretes synovial fluid. They reduce friction where ligaments and tendons pass over bone. Inflammation of a bursa (bursitis) can be idiopathic, due to injury, infection or gout, or part of a systemic inflammatory disease. Some types are notifiable industrial disorders (e.g. coal miner's 'beat' knee).

Olecranon bursitis and prepatellar bursitis are common and their clinical features and management are discussed below.

Olecranon bursitis

This can be precipitated by excessive friction on the elbow, for example students who rest their elbows on desks. Septic olecranon bursitis causes pain on elbow flexion. Idiopathic and traumatic cases are usually only painful when pressure is applied to the bursa. Movement of the elbow is not usually uncomfortable or impaired. On examination the bursa is distended and tender.

Bursal fluid should be aspirated to exclude infection and improve symptoms. Local corticosteroid injection is effective in non-septic cases. A compressive bandage can help recurrence of swelling. Infection should be treated with appropriate antibiotics.

Soft tissue lesions are commonly precipitated by overuse injuries. It is therefore important to ask patients about their work and leisure activities.

Prepatellar or infrapatellar bursitis (housemaid's or carpet-fitter's knee)

This is common in people such as carpet fitters who spend a lot of time kneeling. A hot, red swelling develops over the front of the patella. Active knee extension is usually quite painful. Infection and gout should be excluded by aspirating fluid. Treatment involves rest. Recurrent episodes may require surgical excision of the bursa. Antibiotic therapy should be given for sepsis.

Dupuytren's contracture

Definition

Dupuytren's contracture is a common condition, characterized by nodular fibrosis of the palmar fascia, which draws one or more fingers into flexion.

Incidence

Before the age of 55, the incidence of Dupuytren's contracture is much higher in men. After this time, it is similar in men and women.

Aetiology

It is commoner in patients with certain medical conditions. These are shown in Figure 24.3.

Clinical features

The ulnar side of the hand, especially the ring and little finger, is most commonly affected. Patients usually complain of inability to extend one or more fingers. There is usually little pain. The fibrosis may remain stable or progress. Progressive cases can result in marked deformity and loss of function, with the finger held in a fixed position curled into the palm.

In early cases, nodules may be felt in the palm or on the palmar surface of the finger. In more advanced cases, flexion at the metacarpophalangeal (MCP) joints is seen (see Fig. 5.2) and the palm of the hand cannot be placed flat on a table (positive table top test).

Management

The most effective treatment is surgery. Partial fasciectomy is the most commonly performed procedure. There is a risk of recurrence postoperatively.

Factors associated with Dupuytren's contracture
Family history of Dupuytren's contracture
Hepatic cirrhosis
Peyronie's disease
Diabetes mellitus
Anticonvulsant therapy

Fig. 24.3 Factors associated with Dupuytren's contracture.

- What does the term 'enthesopathy' mean?
- What are the clinical signs of tennis elbow?
- What causes 'triggering' of a finger?
- What conditions are associated with Dupuytren's contracture?

Further reading

Hazleman B, Riley G, and Speed C (eds) 2004 *Soft Tissue Rheumatology*. Oxford Universtiy Press, Oxford

25. Taking a History

Good history taking is a valuable skill. It is very important to establish a good rapport with the patient. Patients who feel comfortable with you will find it easier to tell you about their symptoms and answer your questions. A relaxed, trusting patient will also be easier to examine.

The first things to document in your history are:
- The patient's name, age, sex and hospital number.
- The patient's occupation and dominant hand.
- The date, time and place of the consultation (e.g. outpatient department, casualty).

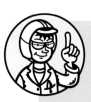 Lesions affecting the dominant hand, wrist, elbow or shoulder will be more disabling than those affecting the non-dominant side.

Presenting complaint

This should be a short statement, summarizing the patient's presenting symptoms. The following are some examples:
- Painful right knee.
- Pain and stiffness of both arms.
- Swollen ankle.

History of the presenting complaint

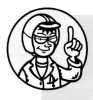 Begin your history with open questions, e.g. 'Tell me about your pain', then ask closed questions if necessary, e.g. 'Does your knee ever give way?'.

This should contain details of the patient's presenting symptoms from their onset to the current time. The following areas should be discussed when taking a rheumatological or orthopaedic history:

Symptom onset
- Date and time of symptom onset.
- Speed of onset—was it acute or gradual?
- Presence of any precipitating factors, such as trauma, commencement of a new drug, etc.

Pain, swelling and stiffness
Establish the following points:
- Site and radiation.
- Nature.
- Periodicity—is it continuous or intermittent?
- Exacerbating and relieving factors.
- Timing—is it worse at any particular time of day?

As a rule, pain and stiffness due to an inflammatory condition such as rheumatoid arthritis are worse first thing in the morning and improve as the day progresses. The duration of the early morning stiffness is quite a good guide to the severity of the inflammation. In contrast, pain due to a mechanical or degenerative problem tends to be worse later in the day, related to exertion and associated with a milder degree of stiffness.

Deformity
Some patients consult their doctor because they have developed a deformity and are concerned. This may or may not be associated with pain. For example, Heberden's nodes due to osteoarthritis can be quite disfiguring, but are not always painful.

Weakness
It is important to ascertain whether this is localized or generalized. Localized weakness suggests a focal problem, such as a peripheral nerve lesion, whereas generalized weakness is more likely to have a systemic cause. True weakness can be myopathic or neurogenic. Sometimes muscle contraction is normal and limited purely by pain.

Numbness
The distribution of numbness or paraesthesia should be documented, as well as any precipitating factors. For example, if numbness affects the radial three and a half fingers, it is probably due to carpal tunnel syndrome. If it affects all the digits, is associated with pallor and provoked by cold weather, Raynaud's phenomenon is more likely.

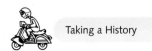

Functional loss and disability

These are common in musculoskeletal disease and can be due to pain, weakness, deformity or any of the other problems discussed above. Loss of function refers to a person's inability to perform an action, such as gripping an object or walking. Disability is the result that functional loss has on that individual's ability to lead a full and active life.

 Always record a patient's level of function in the notes. It is a good marker of progress.

Any restriction that a patient's disease has on the activities of daily living (ADL) should be assessed for two reasons. Firstly, the occupational therapists and other members of the multidisciplinary team may help the patient to find ways of overcoming, or adapting to, the disability. Secondly, a change in the patient's level of function may signify a change in the severity of the disease.

A patient with proximal muscle pain due to polymyalgia rheumatica (PMR) may be unable to rise from a chair at his first clinic visit. When he returns after a month of corticosteroid treatment and jumps out of his chair, you can be fairly confident that he is improving.

Past medical history

Ask about all current and previous medical and surgical disorders, including any musculoskeletal problems. In certain situations, it is worth asking about specific illnesses. For example, a patient with carpal tunnel syndrome may have underlying hypothyroidism or diabetes mellitus.

Drug history

The drug history is always important, but it sometimes has great relevance to orthopaedic and rheumatological problems. Acute gout can be precipitated by the initiation of diuretic therapy, and long-term corticosteroid use can cause osteoporosis.

Social history

Record relevant information about the patient's domestic situation, degree of independence, smoking and alcohol intake.

Family history

Ask particularly about a family history of musculoskeletal disease.

Systemic enquiry

This should include a brief review of any symptoms affecting other systems of the body. It is particularly relevant if you think the patient might have a connective tissue disease.

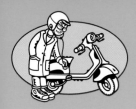

26. General Principles of Examining Joints

Getting off to the right start

It is important to establish a rapport with the patient and you should look smart and be polite!

Always remember to introduce yourself and start by asking if any area is painful before you touch the patient. The last thing you want to do is hurt the patient! There are also specific marks for these acts of courtesy in the Objective Structured Clinical Examination (OSCE).

It is a cliché but the examination really *does* start when the patient enters the room. One of the first things to notice is how the patient walks. Pathological gait patterns are shown in Figure 26.1. Also note how the patient enters the room. The patient could be in a wheelchair, use a stick or walk unaided.

Watch how reliant patients are on relatives during simple tasks such as getting undressed or getting up from a chair.

As soon as you see the patient you should be making a mental note of any features on inspection such as typical features of rheumatoid arthritis in the hands.

Start your examination as you normally would, by looking at the hands first and then moving to the face and so on. Often the majority of features are normal, as in the case of a single osteoarthritic joint.

A thorough general examination is required for patients presenting with:

- Polyarthritis—these patients may have an inflammatory arthropathy, and a general examination is tailored towards looking for extra-articular manifestations. Examination of the cardiovascular system, respiratory system and abdomen is required.
- Widespread aches and pains—these patients may have an inflammatory arthritis, connective tissue disorder or malignancy. Examination of other systems is required such as the skin, eyes and other joints.

Examining joints

- Start with adequate exposure.
- Stand and walk the patient.
- Position the patient for the joint to be examined. Make the patient comfortable and make sure you can get to the correct side of the patient.

When examining joints make sure you stand on the side of the joint to be examined. Don't lean across the patient to examine the opposite hip or knee. A really nasty examiner might put the couch up against the wall and ask you to examine the knee that is beside the wall. If this happens move the couch to the centre of the room!

Pathological patterns of gait		
Gait	**Features**	**Cause**
Trendelenburg	Waddling gait	Loss of abductor function
Antalgic (painful)	The patient tries to offload the painful limb by quickening and shortening the weight-bearing stance phase of the gait cycle	Any painful condition
Short leg gait	Dipping of shoulder on affected side	Any condition causing significant leg length discrepancy
High stepping	Knee is flexed and foot is lifted high to avoid foot dragging on the floor	Nerve palsy (peroneal or sciatic)
Stiff knee	Knee cleared of floor by swinging out away from the body	Fusion of knee

Fig. 26.1 Pathological patterns of gait.

173

- LOOK:
  —Swelling, muscle wasting, scars, erythema, sinus or discharge.
- FEEL:
  —Palpate the joint systematically, noting any effusion and any tenderness over the joint line or other prominent features of the joint.
- MOVE:
  —Demonstrate joint movement actively and passively.
- Any special tests to remember?
- Examine the joints above and below.
- Don't forget peripheral pulses.

Practice a routine on your friends.

Using these basic principles of examining joints you can examine any joint.
For example if asked you *could* examine the temporomandibular joint (I don't expect you to be able to do it) by applying the basic rules.

Examination of the hip

Hip disease is common and examination involves the use of a few special tests that often cause confusion. Unlike with other joints the special tests are used first when examining the hip.

> As a general principle always examine the joints above and below.
> Remember to examine the peripheral vascular system.

Gait

A Trendelenburg gait (waddling) is due to failure of the hip abductors to elevate the pelvis on weight bearing, causing a dipping or rolling gait. To compensate for this the trunk is swung over the weight-bearing hip, which maintains balance.

Failure of hip abduction can be due to pain or ineffectual muscle function following hip surgery (see Fig. 27.1).

The patient may also have an antalgic gait (see Fig. 26.1, p. 173).

Trendelenburg's test

This is used to assess the function of the hip abductors.

Stand behind the patient, expose the pelvis and ask an assistant to stand in front of the patient and hold the patient's hands to prevent a fall. The patient stands on one leg (the leg to be examined remains on the floor) and when hip abductors are functioning the pelvis tilts upwards (Fig. 27.1A and C).

If the abductors are not functioning the pelvis tilts downwards towards the unsupported leg (Fig. 27.1B and D).

Thomas' test

This is a test for fixed flexion of the hip.

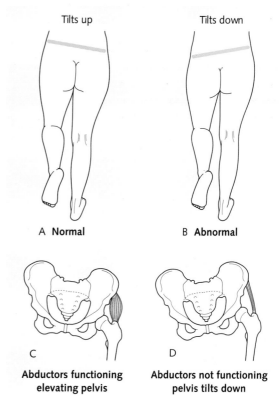

A **Normal** B **Abnormal**

C Abductors functioning elevating pelvis

D Abductors not functioning pelvis tilts down

Fig. 27.1 The Trendelenburg test.

The idea of the test is to abolish the natural lumbar lordosis of the spine and visualize the true degree of flexion deformity at the hip.

To perform the test, the patient is positioned supine (flat on the back) and the opposite hip is flexed fully. This manoeuvre fully corrects the lordosis that is felt by placing a hand under the spine. Now simply observe the degree (if any) of hip flexion (Fig. 27.2).

Leg length discrepancy

Ensure the patient is lying comfortably on the examination couch with the knees straight.

Measure both limbs from the anterior superior iliac spine to the medial malleolus and compare the values.

An idea of where any leg length discrepancy lies can be obtained by flexing both hips and knees and

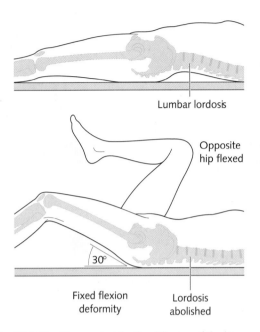

Lumbar lordosis

Opposite hip flexed

30°

Fixed flexion deformity

Lordosis abolished

Fig. 27.2 The Thomas test for fixed flexion of the hip.

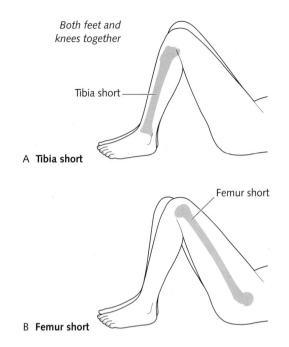

Both feet and knees together

Tibia short

A **Tibia short**

Femur short

B **Femur short**

Fig. 27.3 Assessing leg length discrepancy.

placing them together. Look from the side and determine the relative positions of the knees.

If one knee is higher than the other then this suggests tibial shortness; however, if one knee lies behind the other it suggests a femoral discrepancy (Fig. 27.3).

Inspection

Scars from previous surgery could be present anteriorly, laterally or medially. Look for erythema, sinuses and muscle wasting. Look at both sides of the hip by turning the patient to the prone position.

Palpation

The hip is deeply situated and few features are palpable.

The greater trochanter is easily felt laterally, over which bursitis may be present.

Movement

Normal movements are shown in Figure 27.4.

When assessing hip movements remember to stabilize the pelvis with a hand to ensure that pelvic tilting does not occur.

Examination of the knee

The knee lies superficially and many landmarks are easily palpable.

Don't forget to examine the hip if asked to examine the knee.

Inspection

Ask the patient to stand and walk, and note any gait abnormality.

Deformities (varus, valgus and fixed flexion) are more obvious on standing.

Look for quadriceps wasting, which can be assessed by measuring the thigh circumference and comparing it with the measurement on the other side.

Localized swelling anteriorly or posteriorly may be visible (remember to inspect the back of the knee—this is easily done with the patient standing).

Note an effusion (which can be seen by loss of normal skin dimples at the joint line), scars, erythema or sinuses.

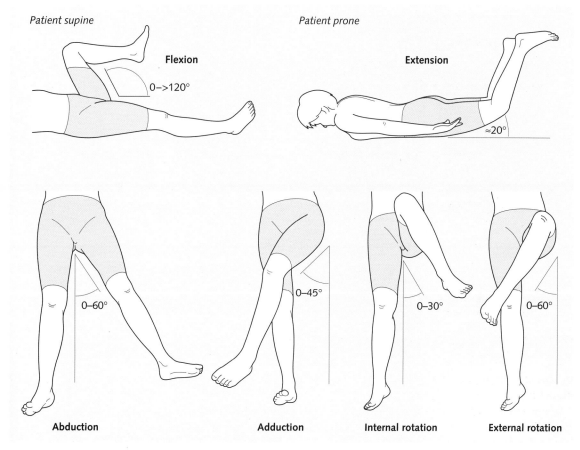

Patient supine

Flexion

0–>120°

Patient prone

Extension

≈20°

Abduction 0–60°

Adduction 0–45°

Internal rotation 0–30°

External rotation 0–60°

Fig. 27.4 Movements of the hip (note all ranges are approximate and vary from patient to patient.

Palpation for an effusion

A knee effusion is important to recognize (Fig. 27.5) as it always indicates pathology. There are two tests commonly used.

Patella tap

Fluid is milked down from the suprapatellar pouch, which lifts the patella away from the femur. The patella is then pushed down onto the femur producing a 'tap' (Fig. 27.6).

Wipe test

Fluid is milked out of the medial dimple. The examining hand then sweeps the fluid from the lateral side of the knee, refilling the medial dimple with a visible bulge.

Palpation

Flexing the knee to 90° allows structures to be palpated more easily.

Be methodical, starting distally over the tibial tubercle and moving proximally, palpating in turn the patellar tendon, proximal tibia, medial and lateral joint lines, femoral condyles, patella, and quadriceps tendon (Fig. 27.7). The collateral ligaments are also palpable (the lateral collateral is a cord-like structure more easily felt with the knee in the figure of four position).

Remember to palpate the posterior aspect of the knee. A Baker's cyst or bursa may be present.

Movement

Both active and passive movement should be tested. The normal range is 0–150° (Fig. 27.8).

Note any fixed flexion or hyperextension of the knee. Feel for patellar crepitus during flexion.

Special tests

Different patients have different degrees of laxity of the ligaments. It is therefore important to compare your examination with the normal side.

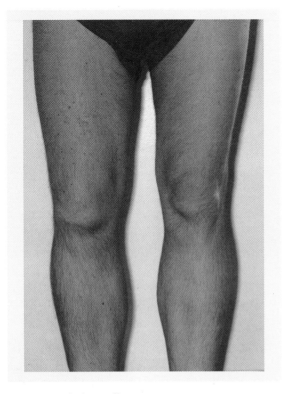

Fig. 27.5 Right knee effusion.

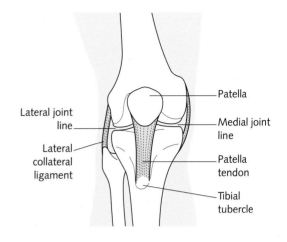

Fig. 27.7 Anatomical structures easily palpated around the knee.

The foot is held between the examiner's elbow and body and both of the examiner's hands are placed on either side of the patient's knee (Fig. 27.9). A valgus or varus strain can then be placed on the knee and opening up of the joint noted.

Collateral ligaments

This test should be performed in full extension and 30° flexion (instability in full extension is *not* present in an isolated ligament rupture and therefore indicates a much more severe injury).

Anterior cruciate ligament (ACL)
Lachman's test

This is the best for ACL deficiency. The idea of the test is to bring the tibia forward on a fixed femur.

Flex the knee to 30°. Then, with the thumbs pointing towards the patient's hip, place one hand

Fig. 27.6 Patella tap sign.

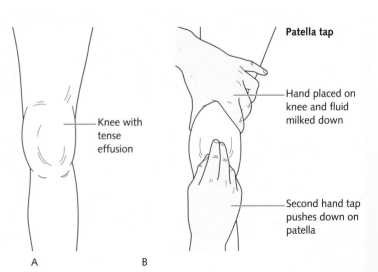

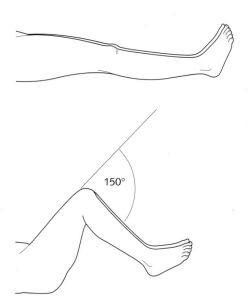

150°

Fig. 27.8 Range of movement of the knee.

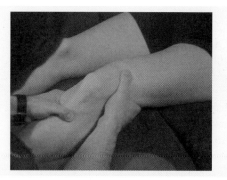

Fig. 27.10 Lachman's test for anterior cruciate ligament deficiency.

around the proximal tibia and stabilize the femur with the other. Lift up on the tibia seeing if there is abnormal forward movement (Fig. 27.10).

Anterior drawer test

This is also a test for ACL deficiency but can be misleading (the anterior drawer test can be positive after medial meniscectomy or in posterior cruciate ligament (PCL) deficiency).

The knee is flexed to 90° and the hamstrings are relaxed. The examiner sits carefully on the patient's foot and both thumbs are placed on the proximal tibia and over both joint lines. The tibia is pulled forward and if movement is excessive the test is positive.

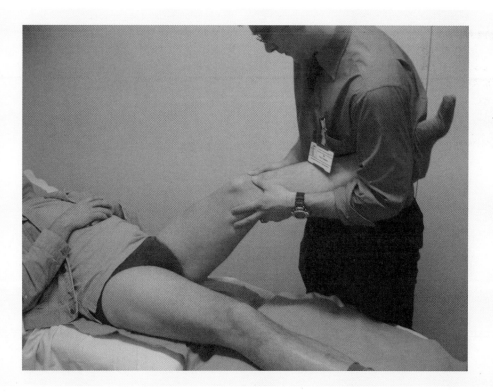

Fig. 27.9 Collateral ligament examination.

Pivot shift test

It can be a difficult test to perform, but the pivot shift is very useful in that it represents the way in which an ACL-deficient knee causes instability and hence gives way.

The test relies on the knee pivoting around the medial collateral ligament and uses the iliotibial band to move the tibia anteriorly.

The flexed knee is held in internal rotation with a valgus force applied as the knee is extended (Fig. 27.11). As the knee comes from flexion to extension at about 15° the tibia jumps forward into a subluxed position.

Posterior cruciate ligament (PCL)

The posterior drawer test is performed exactly as the anterior drawer but the knee is pushed backwards.

The classic sign for a PCL rupture is the posterior sag. This is demonstrated by flexing both knees to 90° and comparing the knee contour (Fig. 27.12). A sag occurs as the tibia falls posteriorly and the tibial tubercle becomes less prominent.

Examining menisci

A variety of tests are performed to assess the integrity of the menisci. None of these tests is

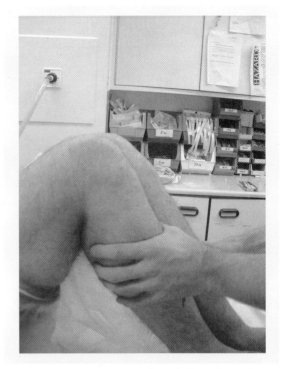

Fig. 27.12 Posterior sag sign. The right knee shows the positive sign. Note that the tibial tuberosity is more prominent on the left.

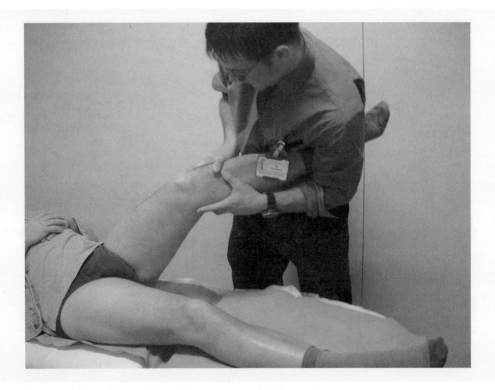

Fig. 27.11 The pivot shift test for instability of the anterior cruciate ligament.

reliable and they are variable depending on the examiner.

The most important clinical finding is joint line tenderness.

The patellofemoral joint

To examine the patellofemoral joint, sit the patient on the edge of the couch so that the legs are free to flex. Watch the patella carefully as the knee extends and look at how the patella tracks. Lateral maltracking is demonstrated as the patella deviates laterally towards the end of extension.

Patella apprehension is demonstrated when the examiner tries to push the patella laterally when the patient's knee is fully extended on the couch. If the patella is unstable the patient will grimace and not let you continue.

Examination of the spine

When examining the spine always remember to also perform a peripheral nervous system examination.

Inspection

In acute conditions muscle spasm and loss of normal lumbar lordosis may be seen. Look at the posture of the patient. If the patient has sciatica the affected leg is often flexed and the patient is stooped.

Note any scars, erythema or deformity. Deformities of the spine such as scoliosis or kyphosis may be obvious on inspection.

- In scoliosis the rib hump deformity is more clearly seen when the patient bends forwards (see Fig. 21.12, p. 152).
- Kyphotic deformity is best visualized from the side (see Fig. 5.4, p. 32). A gibbus is a very pronounced kyphotic deformity caused by fracture, tumour or infection.

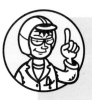

Remember the spine normally has a lumbar and cervical lordosis and a thoracic kyphosis.

Palpation

Palpation is performed standing and with the patient lying prone.

The C7 spinous process is a useful landmark (the most prominent in the upper spine).

Tenderness is elicited by palpation over the spinous processes.

Movement
Cervical spine

Movements of the cervical spine (Fig. 27.13) are usually stated as percentage loss when compared with normal, if possible.

Flexion

Ask the patient to bend the head forward to put the chin on the chest.

Extension

Ask the patient to look up at the ceiling.

Lateral flexion

Ask the patient to put the ear down to the shoulder.

Rotation

Ask the patient to look to either side.

Thoracolumbar spine (Fig. 27.14)
Flexion

Often patients are reluctant to flex the spine if it is acutely tender. Ask patients to bend over and reach as far as they can.

Look and feel for unfolding of the lumbar spine. This can be measured by marking two points on the lumbar spine and observing the increase in the distance between them on flexion.

Extension

Get the patient to arch the back backwards. In conditions such as spinal stenosis this can exacerbate the pain.

Rotation

Stabilize the pelvis by asking the patient to sit when examining rotation in order to abolish hip rotation.

Lateral flexion

Ask the patient to slide one hand down the side of the leg.

Special tests
Straight leg raising

This is a test for nerve root irritation (radiculopathy).

With the patient supine elevate the affected leg passively keeping it straight. If the patient complains of pain down the leg look at the angle that the leg makes with the couch, e.g. 30°. The next step is to

Fig. 27.13 Movements of the cervical spine.

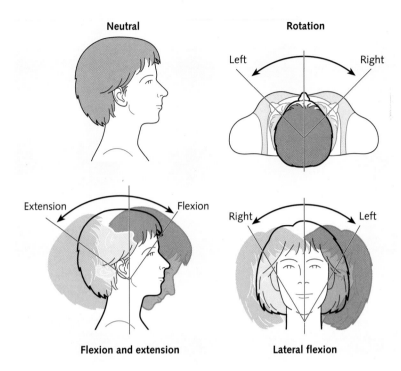

bend the knee as this will abolish the symptoms by relieving tension on the nerve.

For the test to be positive the pain must radiate to the foot (often patients will complain of back pain when elevating the leg).

The crossover sign is present with severe acute prolapsed discs and occurs when the normal leg is elevated causing pain radiating down the opposite leg.

Peripheral nervous examination
Spinal cord conditions such as stenosis or prolapsed disc can cause abnormalities of the peripheral nervous system due to compression on nerve roots. The most commonly affected are the L5 and S1 nerve roots.

Lower limb
Tone
Lower limb tone is usually normal but is reduced in spinal cord compression (flaccid paralysis).

Power is assessed by Medical Research Council (MRC) grade:

0 Nothing.
1 Flicker.
2 Power to move limb with gravity eliminated.
3 Power to move limb against gravity.
4 Reduced from normal.
5 Normal.

Test muscle function as shown in Figure 27.15.

Reflexes
Always compare the reflexes with the opposite limb and make sure the patient is relaxed. Reflexes can be reduced, brisk or absent.

Three reflexes are commonly tested:

- Knee L3–L4: flex both knees over the couch and tap lightly on the patellar ligament.
- Ankle L5, S1: dorsiflex the ankle with the knees flexed and the leg externally rotated. Tap the Achilles tendon.
- Plantar: this is performed by stroking the plantar skin with the handle of the tendon hammer. If the toes extend this is abnormal and called 'up going', indicating an upper motor neuron lesion.

Sensation
Ask the patient if the sensation is normal and the same as on the other side. Dermatomes are shown in Figure 27.16.

Anal tone
In cauda equina syndrome anal tone is lost; therefore an examination per rectum (PR) is an important part of any spinal examination.

Perianal sensation
This is also reduced in cauda equina syndrome.

Fig. 27.14 Thoracolumbar movements.

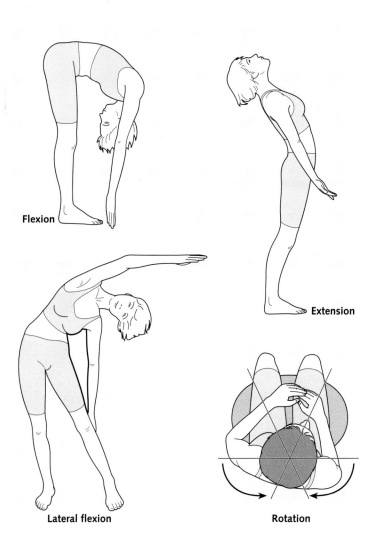

Flexion

Extension

Lateral flexion

Rotation

Testing lower limb muscle function (myotomes)	
Muscle action	Nerve roots tested
Hip flexion (iliopsoas)	L1, L2
Knee flexion (quadriceps)	L3
Ankle dorsiflexion (tibialis anterior)	L4
Great toe extension (extensor hallucis longus)	L5
Ankle plantar flexion (soleus/gastrocnemius)	S1

Fig. 27.15 Testing lower limb muscle function.

Chest expansion

Patients with severe scoliosis or ankylosing spondylitis have reduced lung function and may show reduced chest expansion.

Movement of the shoulder occurs at four joints (Fig. 27.17). The majority of the total range of movement arises from the glenohumeral and scapulothoracic joints. The acromioclavicular and sternoclavicular joints contribute very little.

Inspection

Look at the position and contours of the shoulder and compare with the opposite one.

- Swelling of the shoulder is uncommon. When it does occur, it is best seen anteriorly.
- Muscle wasting may be due to chronic shoulder pathology, such as chronic rotator cuff tendinitis.

Palpation

Feel for tenderness and swelling of the acromioclavicular, sternoclavicular and glenohumeral joints. A gap on palpation of the acromioclavicular joint indicates dislocation. Crepitus of the glenohumeral or acromioclavicular joints may be felt on shoulder movement. Palpate the muscles of the shoulder girdle and neck to identify any tender 'trigger' points of fibromyalgia (see Fig. 17.3, p. 124).

Movement

Examine active and passive movements, looking at the range of abduction, forward flexion, and internal and external rotation.

- A normal range of passive movements suggests that glenohumeral disease is very unlikely.
- Normal passive movements with painful or restricted active movements indicate a muscle or tendon problem.
- A 'hitch-up' of the shoulder on active abduction of the arm is a sign of reduced glenohumeral range (Fig. 27.18).
- Loss of passive external rotation, with 'hitching' and abduction limited to 90° are highly indicative of a capsular lesion, as in adhesive capsulitis ('frozen shoulder').

A quick way to evaluate active shoulder movements is by asking patients to:

- Put their hands behind their head, with the elbows back.
- Reach behind their back, as if to fasten a bra strap.
- Raise their arms up to their sides and then above their head.

The rotator cuff

The supraspinatus, infraspinatus, teres minor and subscapularis muscles make up the rotator cuff. They hold the head of the humerus in the glenoid cavity, maintain stability and initiate shoulder abduction. Rotator cuff inflammation, injury and degeneration are common. Disease of the supraspinatus especially, causes pain on abduction when the tendon becomes compressed under the acromion. The pain is felt at between 60° and 120° of abduction (Fig. 27.19). This is referred to as a 'painful arc'.

Resisted shoulder movement should be examined. Pain or weakness on resisted movement suggests involvement of the rotator cuff muscles and tendons.

- Supraspinatus is tested with the arm abducted to 90°, flexed to 30° and internally rotated with the

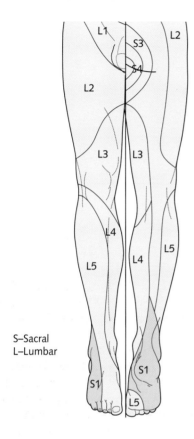

S–Sacral
L–Lumbar

Fig. 27.16 Dermatomes of the lower limb.

- Rupture of the long head of biceps is usually obvious, as it produces a bulge anteriorly in the upper arm.
- Look for winging of the scapula by asking the patient to do a press-up against the wall. Weakness of the serratus anterior muscle causes the medial border to protrude backwards. This can occur in long thoracic nerve palsy or other causes of muscular weakness.
- Look for a step in the acromioclavicular joint due to dislocation. This is seen best whilst the patient's arm is hanging in a relaxed position.

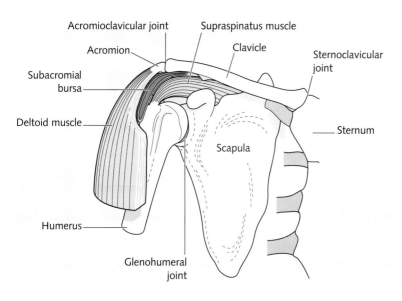

Fig. 27.17 Anatomy of the shoulder.

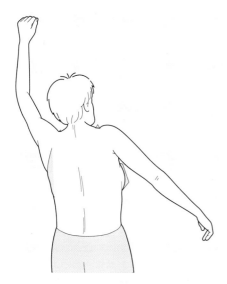

Fig. 27.18 A 'hitched' shoulder. The patient is unable to elevate her arm to the side properly, so is 'cheating' by shrugging her shoulder.

thumb pointing downwards. Abduction is then resisted.
- Resisted internal rotation tests the subscapularis.
- Resisted external rotation tests the infraspinatus and teres minor.

Apprehension testing

An unstable shoulder makes the patient apprehensive when it is put into abduction and external rotation.

The patient should be supine with the arms abducted to 90° and elbows flexed to 90°. Ask the patient to lower the hands backward (i.e. towards 90° of external rotation.) The patient's apprehension will limit external rotation of a dislocation-prone shoulder. This position is also useful for detecting subtle abnormalitites of shoulder movement that you have not detected in the other ways described—look for asymmetry in the degree to which the patient is able to rotate the shoulder externally in this position.

Acromioclavicular joint testing

Pain arising from pathology of the acromioclavicular joint may be accentuated if the patient places the hand on the opposite shoulder and the examiner pulls the elbow in the same direction. If a step in the acromioclavicular joint is observed, try returning the acromion to its normal position by stabilizing the clavicle with one hand and lifting the elbow with the other.

Examination of the elbow

The elbow joint consists of two articulations:
- The first is between the humerus, radius and ulna, which allows flexion to a range of 150°.
- The second is the superior radioulnar joint, which allows rotation of the wrist through 180°.

185

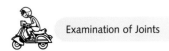

Fig. 27.19 Demonstration of the painful arc.

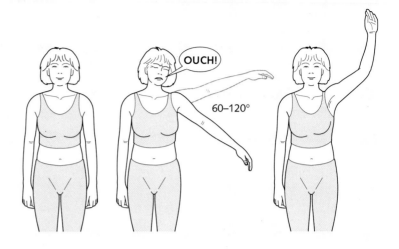

Inspection

Inspect the elbow from behind with the patient's arm flexed and extended. The lateral infracondylar recess will be filled in if an effusion is present. Look also for swelling of the olecranon bursa and the presence of rheumatoid nodules along the border of the ulna.

Palpation

Palpate the olecranon process and medial and lateral epicondyles. The lateral epicondyle will be tender in tennis elbow. The radial head is usually felt easily in the lateral aspect of the joint and its movement can be assessed during pronation and supination.

Movement

Test flexion, extension, pronation and supination. Extension of the elbow is to 180° or beyond in almost all normal people. The inability to straighten the elbow to 180° is therefore considered pathological, even if it is pain-free and unnoticed by the patient. It will usually be a sign of arthritis and may support this diagnosis in a patient giving a history of episodic joint pain. On the other hand, many people can extend another 5–10°. So hyperextension (as in hypermobility) is defined as extension beyond 190°.

It is best to assess pronation and supination with the elbow flexed to 90° and held close to the side of the body. If you suspect the patient may have epicondylitis, examine resisted movements of the wrist for pain (see Fig. 24.1, p. 165).

Examination of the wrist and hand

Inspection

Inspection of the hands is an important part of the musculoskeletal examination. Look first at the skin and the nails.

- Pitting of the nails or onycholysis is commonly found in psoriatic arthritis.
- Nail fold infarcts and digital ulcers can occur as a consequence of vasculitis. A magnifying glass is useful when looking for nail fold infarcts.
- Telangiectasia and sclerodactyly are features of systemic sclerosis.
- Heberden's nodes, gouty tophi or rheumatoid nodules may develop in the fingers.

Look next for deformities, which are common in inflammatory arthritis. Arthritis mutilans is a rare, but severe type of joint destruction in psoriatic arthritis. Rheumatoid arthritis (RA) can cause many deformities in the hand and wrist, including:

- Volar subluxation and radial deviation of the carpus.
- Boutonnière and swan-neck deformities of the fingers (see Fig. 9.9, p. 54).
- Z-deformity of the thumb.

Look carefully for swelling. The distribution gives a good clue to the cause. For example, swelling of the metacarpophalangeal (MCP) and proximal interphalangeal (PIP) joints is common in RA, whereas distal interphalangeal (DIP) joint involvement is more typical of osteoarthritis (OA) or psoriatic arthritis. The swelling of tenosynovitis follows the route of the tendon.

It is also important to note any muscle wasting. Atrophy of the dorsal interossei occurs in RA. Carpal tunnel syndrome can lead to wasting of the muscles of the thenar eminence.

Palpation

Palpate any swellings to confirm whether they are hard due to bony overgrowth, or soft due to synovitis. Synovitis at the MCP joints is best felt with the patient's fingers semi-flexed and the examiner's fingertips placed at either side of the MCP joint, feeling for soft tissue swelling. With practice, it is easily detected, even in podgy hands. Synovitis at the PIP joint bulges out either side of the extensor expansion. Enthesitis at the DIP joint of psoriatic arthritis or Reiter's syndrome is to be distinguished from Heberden's nodes; this is not always easy. Crepitus, often with pain, may be felt on palpation of the first carpometacarpal (CMC) joint in OA. Tenosynovitis of the finger flexors can be associated with tendon nodules, which can be felt moving on finger flexion.

Movement

It is important to assess hand function. Active and passive movement of the wrist and digits should be tested, as well as the patient's ability to perform certain tasks. The muscles responsible for various movements of the hand and wrist are shown in Figure 27.20.

The 'prayer' sign is useful when assessing hand and wrist function. Ask the patient to extend both wrists and place the palms of the hands flat against each other, as if praying (Fig. 27.21). Patients with limited wrist extension or deformities or synovitis of their MCP or PIP joints will find this difficult.

 Ask the patient to pick a penny up from the table or fasten a button. This will give you a good idea of what the patient's hand function is like. It is surprising how well some people can perform fiddly tasks, despite having hand deformities.

Special tests

Tinel's and Phalen's tests should be performed in patients who have symptoms suggestive of carpal

Fig. 27.20 Muscles responsible for hand and wrist movement.

Muscles responsible for hand and wrist movement	
Movement	**Muscle(s) responsible (nerve supply)**
Wrist flexion	Flexor carpi radialis (median) Flexor carpi ulnaris (ulnar) Palmaris longus (median)
Wrist extension	Extensor carpi radialis longus and brevis (both radial) Extensor carpi ulnaris (radial)
DIP joint flexion	Flexor digitorum profundus (median and ulnar)
PIP joint flexion	Flexor digitorum superficialis (median)
MCP joint flexion and IP joint extension	Lumbricals (median and ulnar)
Finger abduction	Dorsal interossei (ulnar)
Finger adduction	Palmar interossei (ulnar)
Extension of MCPs, PIPs and DIPs	Extensor digitorum (radial)
Thumb abduction	Abductor pollicis brevis (median)
Thumb adduction	Adductor pollicis (ulnar)
Thumb opposition	Opponens pollicis (median)
Thumb extension	Extensor pollicis longus (radial)

21/10/03

New patient
9.30am admitted via A+E
History from patient and daughter

Mrs A Moore   DOB 16/9/27
76 year old lady retired teacher

> 1. Presenting complaint should be brief, but it is helpful to mention relevant background information.

PC   Found on floor
            C/O pain right hip

HOPC   Patient found on floor by relative
            Fall last night at home in the kitchen
            Unable to get up due to sudden pain right hip
            Severe constant pain in right groin
            °radiation
            Aggravated by movement / no relieving factors
            Unable to move right leg
            On floor overnight and found by worried
            relative in morning
            Fall due to dizzy spell
            No loss of consciousness, no chest pain

> 2. Establish cause of fall. Simple trip or medical problem?

PMH   °DM, ° asthma, °epilepsy, °MI, °CVA, °RhF
            Mild hypertension
            Tonsillectomy aged 14
            Hysterectomy aged 50

> 3. Always record the dose and frequency of any drugs – remember you'll be writing the drug chart later! Always document that you have asked about drug allergies

DH   Frusemide 20mg od
            Atenolol 50mg od
            Aspirin 75mg od
            °allergies

SH   Widow
            Lives alone in ground floor flat
            Independent
            Does own shopping, cooking and housework
            Daughter visits regularly
            Non-smoker
            Alcohol at Xmas only
FH   No family history of illness

SE

CVS   No chest pain / palpitations / orthopnoea / intermittent claudication / ankle oedema
RS   No cough / haemoptysis / wheeze / S.O.B.
GI   No change in bowel habit / PR bleeding / indigestion / abdominal pains
GU   No dysuria / haematuria / frequency / urgency
CNS   No headaches / fits / paraesthesia
            previous dizzy spells ×2
MS   Mild arthritis both knees

Fig. 28.2 Orthopaedic clerking

O/E   Alert and oriented in pain
          AMT 10/10   °A °C °C °L

> **4.** Record your initial observations – they are important. 'Alert & chatty' or 'distressed & looks unwell' tell you a lot about the patient.

CVS   Pulse 90 regular
         BP 130/85
         JVP →
         HS I + II o nil added
         Peripheral pulses present
         slight ankle oedema
RS   Resp rate 20/min-shallow
         Trachea central
         Chest expansion R=L
         AE equal
         Breath sounds vesicular nil added
         °ankle oedema

AS   soft non-tender
       °masses °liver °spleen okidneys
       BS ✓
       HO ✓
       Femoral pulses palpable
       Hysterectomy scar

> **5.** Always use diagrams to clarify your examination findings.

Musculoskeletal system
Right leg shortened and externally rotated
Unable to assess movement due to pain
Skin ✓ pulse ✓ toes ✓ sensation ✓

CNS   Cranial nerves intact
        Tone, power, reflexes and sensation equal
        and normal (difficult to assess right leg
        formally due to pain)

> **6.** If there is no abnormality of the CNS, simply include a one-line summary.

Impression A 76-year-old lady who is normally well and independent
         with a history of an unwitnessed collapse resulting in pain
         and deformity of the right leg

Differential diagnosis
      1 Fracture right neck of femur secondary to
        collapse ?cause
      2 dehydration secondary to being
        on floor overnight
      3 ?? CVA

Investigations
      FBC, V+E, glucose, LFTs, Ca prof, TFTs, cardiac enzymes
      ECG, CXR
      X-ray right hip confirms displaced intra-capsular hip fracture

Management plan
Admit
Analgesia
IV fluids
Monitor fluid input and output / catheterize patient
Distal and general observations
DVT prophylaxis
Needs medical opinion re collapse ?cause contact med Reg
For theatre when fit
needs consent for hemiarthroplasty (registrar informed)
NBM from midnight
For discussion at trauma meeting tomorrow, will need anaesthetic review

> **7.** Always include a management plan – even when you are still a student. It might not be right but you need to start training yourself to think like a doctor.

> **8.** Sign your notes, including printed surname and bleep number.

HASLAM 562

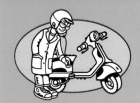

29. Investigations

Blood tests

The following blood tests are useful in the investigation of rheumatic disease.

Full blood count

Chronic inflammatory disease can cause anaemia, but the haemoglobin rarely drops below 9 g/dL.

- Anaemia may be due to chronic disease or iron deficiency from non-steroidal anti-inflammatory drug (NSAID) therapy.
- A polymorphonuclear leucocytosis may be a consequence of infection, such as septic arthritis or osteomyelitis. It can also be a sign of inflammation or prolonged corticosteroid use.
- Leucopenia can be a feature of systemic lupus erythematosus (SLE) or bone marrow suppression from disease-modifying antirheumatic drugs (DMARDs).
- Thrombocytosis often occurs in active inflammatory disease. It is sometimes referred to as a 'reactive thrombocytosis'.

Erythrocyte sedimentation rate (ESR) and C-reactive protein (CRP)

- These are non-specific markers of inflammation and will rise in infectious and inflammatory disorders.
- The ESR measures aggregation of erythrocytes, which increases with the concentration of plasma proteins such as fibrinogen and immunoglobulins.
- The upper limit of normal for the ESR increases with age.
- CRP is synthesized by the liver and rises within 6–10 hours of an inflammatory event.

The CRP responds more rapidly than the ESR to inflammation.

Urea and electrolytes (U&E)

Renal impairment might occur in gout or connective tissue disease.

Liver function tests (LFTs)

- A raised level of alkaline phosphatase is seen in Paget's disease.
- Many drugs used for musculoskeletal problems can be hepatotoxic, such as methotrexate and NSAIDs.

Uric acid

- Prolonged hyperuricaemia predisposes to gout.
- Occasionally, uric acid levels are normal during an acute attack of gout.

Calcium

- Hypocalcaemia occurs in osteomalacia.
- Hypercalcaemia can be a feature of malignancy.

Creatine kinase (CK)

- This muscle enzyme exists as three isoenzymes (CK-MM, CK-MB and CK-BB).
- Elevated levels of CK-MM may be due to myositis or other causes of skeletal muscle damage.
- CK-BB is found in the brain and CK-MB in the myocardium.

Autoantibodies

These are found in many autoimmune rheumatic diseases. Medical students and doctors often find the results of autoantibody tests difficult to interpret, but this is usually because the tests have been requested inappropriately. Some autoantibodies can occur in healthy people and tests for them have little diagnostic value unless they are done in appropriate circumstances.

Example

An elderly man visits his doctor complaining of pain in his knees that is worse in the evenings and has been present for several years. On examination, he has bilateral knee crepitus, without swelling and Heberden's and Bouchard's nodes in his hands. His family doctor requests several investigations, including a test for rheumatoid factor, which is positive. There is now confusion as to the correct

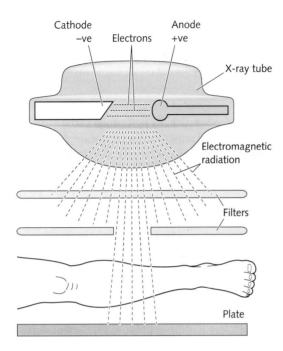

Fig. 29.3 Production of a radiographic image.

Two views are required, taken at 90° to each other, of the joint or bone to be examined (usually anteroposterior (AP) and lateral). Sometimes special views are taken, such as scaphoid views when looking for a fracture.

Fluoroscopy (also known as screening) uses the same principles as radiography but the image is obtained on a screen and is in real time (i.e. moving). Screening is commonly used intraoperatively in orthopaedic surgery when fixing fractures and as guidance for joint injections.

Ultrasound

Ultrasound is used widely in orthopaedics and has the advantages of being cheap, portable and safe, and it allows dynamic images.

The image is produced using a transducer that emits a beam of high-frequency sound (ultrasound) and detects the sound waves reflected from the soft tissues of the patient. Different tissues absorb or reflect different amounts of the sound beam, and the reflections are analysed to produce a black and white image.

Areas commonly imaged in this way include the shoulder for rotator cuff tears, the hip for joint effusion, and extra-articular structures around the knee such as the patellar tendon.

Ultrasound can also be used for guidance, for example for joint aspiration.

Computed tomography (CT)

CT uses the basic principles of an X-ray machine but the image is obtained when the X-ray tube is circled around the patient in the scanner. Instead of an X-ray plate the CT scanner has detectors within the machine to collect images. A large number of images are acquired and processed by the computer and the resulting images are in the form of cross-sectional slices taken in different planes.

The main role for CT in orthopaedics is the study of bones, particularly complex fractures.

Remember that CT scans also produce a significant radiation exposure.

It is also possible to reconstruct images in three dimensions. Three-dimensional (3-D) reconstructions are useful in orthopaedics when planning complex pelvic or hip surgery.

Magnetic resonance imaging (MRI)

MRI gives excellent images of soft tissues and bone marrow.

The images are generated by the use of a powerful magnet, which aligns protons in the body with the electromagnetic field. A pulse of radiofrequency energy then causes the protons to 'flip' (change alignment) and images are acquired when energy is released as the protons realign themselves within the magnetic field. A coil collects data, which are then reconstructed with complex computer software to produce the image.

As a large magnet is used, any metal components or foreign bodies may become dislodged. Patients with cardiac pacemakers and intraocular metallic foreign bodies must not have an MRI scan.

MRI is commonly used around the knee to look for meniscal or ligamentous injuries (Fig. 29.4), the shoulder for capsule or rotator cuff lesions, and the spine for disc prolapse and nerve root compression.

MRI is also good at assessing bone changes such as in infection, tumour and osteonecrosis.

Isotope bone scan

An isotope bone scan involves the use of a radioactive tracer injected intravenously and taken up by physiologically active bone. The most commonly used is technetium-99m (^{99m}Tc) and its decay is measured with a gamma camera. The procedure is divided into three phases depending on the time

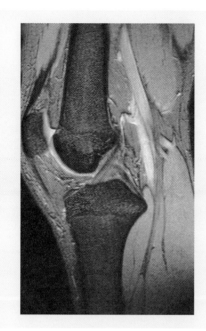

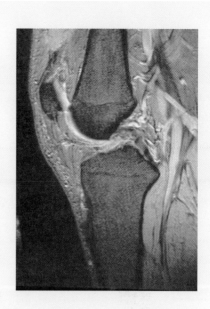

Fig. 29.4 MRI scans of the knee: (A) normal; (B) showing rupture of both cruciate ligaments.

after injection: blood flow (initial); blood pool (30 minutes); and delayed (4 hours).

The images obtained show an outline of the body with areas highlighted where the isotope has accumulated.

Bone scans are useful as a tool for identifying the presence of a disease process (sensitive) but not very good at telling you exactly what the disease is (non-specific). Increased uptake occurs typically in growth plates, arthritis, fractures, metastases (commonly used in malignancy), infection and Paget's disease. Decreased uptake occurs in some tumours (haemopoietic) and also in avascular bone.

Dual energy X-ray absorptiometry (DEXA)

This is the procedure of choice for the diagnosis of osteoporosis and for determining subsequent fracture risk.

Measurement of bone density is made at the hip and compared with control values.

Arthrography

Arthrograms are investigations in which the patient also has contrast or air injected into the joint. Plain X-ray arthrograms have largely been superseded by other investigations but are still used for hip conditions in the child. CT and MRI arthrograms are now becoming widespread for the diagnosis of intra-articular pathology, particularly in the shoulder such as a Bankart lesion.

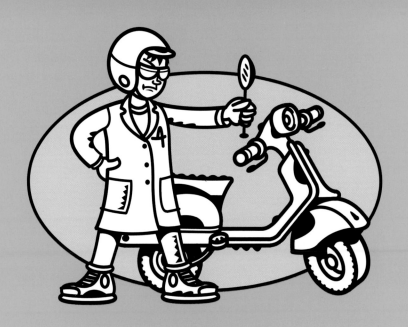

SELF-ASSESSMENT

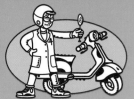
Indicate whether each answer is true or false.

Rheumatology

1. Rheumatoid arthritis:

(a) Is associated with the HLA-DR4 genotype.
(b) Rarely affects the hands.
(c) Affects women more commonly than it affects men.
(d) Is a disease that only affects the joints.
(e) Only occurs in people who have a positive serum rheumatoid factor.

2. Gout:

(a) Is more common in people with a low body mass index.
(b) Is a recognized cause of renal failure.
(c) Often causes X-ray changes after the first attack.
(d) Can be caused by high-dose salicylate therapy.
(e) Commonly affects the first metatarsophalangeal (MTP) joint.

3. The following features are recognized complications of ankylosing spondylitis:

(a) Atlantoaxial subluxation.
(b) Mitral stenosis.
(c) Plantar fasciitis.
(d) Anterior uveitis.
(e) Pulmonary fibrosis.

4. Psoriatic arthropathy:

(a) Affects over 50% of people with psoriasis.
(b) May precede the development of psoriatic skin lesions.
(c) Tends to worsen in parallel with the skin disease.
(d) Often causes dactylitis.
(e) Does not cause erosions.

5. Sjögren's syndrome:

(a) Is characterized by inflammation of endocrine glands.
(b) Is associated with an increase in autoantibody production.
(c) Can occur in patients with rheumatoid arthritis.
(d) Can affect the nervous system.
(e) Is associated with the development of carcinomas.

6. Giant cell arteritis (GCA):

(a) Is always associated with a high erythrocyte sedimentation rate (ESR).
(b) Rarely affects the elderly.
(c) Can cause blindness.
(d) Can always be diagnosed with a temporal artery biopsy.
(e) Can occur in association with polymyalgia rheumatica (PMR).

7. Fibromyalgia:

(a) Affects men more commonly than it affects women.
(b) Causes joint inflammation.
(c) Is commonly associated with anxiety and depression.
(d) Causes soft tissue tenderness.
(e) Is usually cured by cognitive behavioural therapy.

8. Systemic lupus erythematosus (SLE):

(a) Can be induced by the drug minocycline.
(b) Often causes erosive damage to the joints.
(c) Is associated with a positive antinuclear antibody in 30–40% of patients.
(d) Only causes a raised erythrocyte sedimentation rate (ESR) if infection, serositis or synovitis is present.
(e) Is a recognized cause of seizures.

9. Dermatomyositis:

(a) Can develop in childhood.
(b) Typically presents with distal muscle weakness.
(c) Is more likely than polymyositis to be associated with an underlying malignancy.
(d) Can cause a rash on the dorsum of the hands.
(e) Causes an elevated creatine kinase.

10. Tennis elbow:

(a) Only develops in tennis players.
(b) Causes tenderness over the medial epicondyle.
(c) Pain is exacerbated by resisted wrist flexion.
(d) May be a feature of enteropathic arthritis.
(e) Often improves with rest.

11. Carpal tunnel syndrome:

(a) Is due to compression of the median nerve.
(b) Causes pain in the ring and little fingers.
(c) May result in weakness of the thenar muscles.
(d) May be associated with diabetes mellitus.
(e) Is a common complication of rheumatoid arthritis.

12. Disease-modifying antirheumatic drugs (DMARDs):

(a) Have a quick onset of action.
(b) Are not usually prescribed in rheumatoid arthritis until patients have developed joint erosions.
(c) Should never be used in conjunction with corticosteroids.
(d) May suppress the immune system.
(e) May cause bone marrow suppression.

13. The following suggest that joint pain is due to an inflammatory cause:

(a) The pain is at its worst first thing in the morning.
(b) The joints feel stiff for at least 30 minutes after rising from bed.
(c) The pain is associated with fatigue.
(d) There is associated 'boggy' swelling of the joints.
(e) The joints feel warm on palpation.

14. The erythrocyte sedimentation rate (ESR):

(a) Measures aggregation of erythrocytes.
(b) Is always raised if the C-reactive protein (CRP) is elevated.
(c) Has a normal range that changes with age.
(d) Is always elevated in cases of inflammatory joint disease.
(e) Increases with the concentration of plasma proteins.

15. Determine whether the following statements regarding radiological investigations are true or false:

(a) The vertebrae become squared in ankylosing spondylitis.
(b) Rheumatoid arthritis causes periarticular sclerosis of bone.
(c) Sclerosis of the sacroiliac joints may be seen in psoriatic arthritis.
(d) Calcification of cartilage in the menisci of the knee is a common feature of pyrophosphate arthropathy.
(e) Magnetic resonance imaging is capable of detecting the bony erosions of rheumatoid arthritis before they are visible on plain X-rays.

16. Reactive arthritis:

(a) Is a form of septic arthritis.
(b) Is often triggered by a genitourinary infection.
(c) Usually affects the joints symmetrically.
(d) Never causes dactylitis.
(e) Can cause symptoms for several months.

17. Determine whether the following statements regarding musculoskeletal deformities are true or false:

(a) Bouchard's nodes are a feature of rheumatoid arthritis.
(b) Ulnar deviation of the wrist occurs in rheumatoid arthritis.
(c) 'Jaccoud's arthritis' is the name used to describe the hand deformities of rheumatoid arthritis.
(d) The 'question-mark' posture in ankylosing spondylitis describes the exaggerated lumbar lordosis and extension of the thoracic and cervical spines.
(e) Arthritis mutilans is a severe deformity seen in the hands of some patients with psoriatic arthritis.

18. Determine whether the following statements regarding the skin in musculoskeletal disease are true or false.

(a) Keratoderma blennorrhagica affects some patients with reactive arthritis.
(b) A 'butterfly' rash is a common feature of systemic sclerosis.
(c) Vasculitis can present with urticarial lesions, ulceration, ischaemia, palpable purpura and splinter haemorrhages.
(d) A lilac-coloured rash of the skin over the eyelids occurs in polymyositis.
(e) Telangiectasia are seen more commonly in limited than in diffuse systemic sclerosis.

19. Dupuytren's contracture:

(a) Occurs more commonly in individuals who have a positive family history of the disease.
(b) Is characterized by nodular fibrosis of the palmar fascia.
(c) Affects the index finger more commonly than it affects the little finger.
(d) Is more common in alcoholics than in people who abstain.
(e) Can recur after surgical treatment.

20. Regarding the antiphospholipid antibody syndrome:

(a) It can present with transient ischaemic attacks.
(b) It can present with migraine.
(c) Female patients with antiphospholipid antibody syndrome should be strongly encouraged to take the combined oral contraceptive pill.
(d) A pregnant woman with the antiphospholipid antibody syndrome and a history of fetal loss should be fully anticoagulated with warfarin throughout her pregnancy.
(e) Serological tests for syphilis (e.g. VDRL) may be falsely positive in patients with lupus anticoagulant or anticardiolipin antibodies.

21. Regarding synovial fluid:

(a) Only infected joints produce cloudy synovial fluid.
(b) Septic arthritis can be confidently excluded if no organisms are seen on microscopy of freshly aspirated synovial fluid.
(c) For accurate identification of crystals, synovial fluid must be examined under a polarized light microscope.
(d) Urate crystals are needle-shaped and show strong negative birefringence.
(e) Calcium pyrophosphate dihydrate (CPPD) crystals are either rhomboid or rod-shaped and show negative birefringence.

22. The following can cause pain in the forefoot:

(a) Morton's neuroma.
(b) Pre-Achilles bursitis.
(c) Hallux rigidus.
(d) Acute gout.
(e) Tarsal tunnel syndrome.

23. Regarding platelets:

(a) Thrombocytopenia can occur in methotrexate toxicity.
(b) Thrombocytopenia can be a feature of systemic lupus erythematosus (SLE).
(c) Thrombocytosis can be a feature of active vasculitis.
(d) Thrombocytosis can be a feature of active rheumatoid arthritis.
(e) The antiphospholipid antibody syndrome causes thrombocytosis.

24. Regarding juvenile idiopathic arthritis:

(a) It can cause growth retardation.
(b) Splinting of joints may help prevent deformity.
(c) Oligoarticular disease affects five or more joints.
(d) Children with enthesitis-related arthritis are often HLA-DR4 positive.
(e) A positive antinuclear antibody is associated with a reduced risk of uveitis.

25. Regarding systemic sclerosis:

(a) It is more common in men than in women.
(b) Raynaud's phenomenon is a common feature.
(c) Gastrointestinal complications are the most frequent cause of death.
(d) Pulmonary hypertension is a recognized complication.
(e) It can involve the myocardium, leading to cardiac failure.

26. Vasculitis:

(a) Is often cured by a short course of low-dose oral corticosteroids.
(b) Can cause infarction due to stenosis of blood vessels.
(c) Can cause haemorrhage due to rupture of blood vessels.
(d) Is rarely symptomatic if it affects small blood vessels.
(e) Can complicate HIV infection.

27. Sensory loss in the foot may be caused by:

(a) Diabetes mellitus.
(b) Plantar fasciitis.
(c) Tarsal tunnel syndrome.
(d) Morton's neuroma.
(e) Achilles tendinitis.

28. The following may be manifestations of systemic lupus erythematosus (SLE):

(a) Fever.
(b) Calcinosis.
(c) Photosensitivity.
(d) Hepatic cirrhosis.
(e) Conjunctivitis.

29. The following are recognized causes of secondary Sjögren's syndrome:

(a) Osteoarthritis.
(b) Paget's disease.
(c) Polymyositis.
(d) Chronic active hepatitis.
(e) Multiple sclerosis.

30. Decide whether the statements below concerning autoantibodies are true or false:

(a) Titres of anti-double-stranded DNA antibodies rise during a flare of rheumatoid arthritis (RA).
(b) Rheumatoid factor antibodies may be detected in patients with primary Sjögren's syndrome.
(c) Antihistone antibodies are associated with drug-induced systemic lupus erythematosus (SLE).
(d) Antibodies to serine proteinase 3 are found in patients with Wegener's granulomatosis.
(e) Antinuclear antibodies are found in 40% of the normal population.

31. The following may be extra-articular features of rheumatoid arthritis (RA):

(a) Anterior uveitis.
(b) Pericarditis.
(c) Pleural effusion.
(d) Hypothyroidism.
(e) Pulmonary fibrosis.

32. Felty's syndrome:

(a) Is an extra-articular manifestation of rheumatoid arthritis.
(b) Causes hepatomegaly.
(c) Is associated with a neutrophil leucocytosis.
(d) Makes patients prone to bacterial infections.
(e) Usually affects patients who are rheumatoid factor negative.

33. Regarding calcium pyrophosphate dihydrate crystals:

(a) They may be deposited in tendons.
(b) They can cause acute gout.
(c) They can cause a chronic arthropathy.
(d) Deposition is more common in patients with haemochromatosis.
(e) They may be detected in synovial fluid that also contains monosodium urate crystals.

14. Osteomalacia:

(a) Results from decreased calcium intake.
(b) Can be diagnosed by Looser's zones on X-ray.
(c) Weakens bony structure.
(d) Is caused by increased activity of osteoblasts.
(e) Is usually treated with vitamin D supplements.

15. Paget's disease of bone:

(a) Can weaken bone, predisposing to pathological fractures.
(b) Presents with bone pain in the majority of patients.
(c) Is treated with bisphosphonates.
(d) Is associated with very vascular bone.
(e) Often produces deformity.

16. Spinal stenosis:

(a) Is due to narrowing of the spinal canal.
(b) Causes symptoms which are worse after walking and relieved by rest.
(c) Is thought to be due to ischaemia of the nerve roots.
(d) Always gives sharp shooting pain into the foot.
(e) Is usually a disease of older men with manual jobs.

17. A lesion in bone on X-ray is likely to be malignant if:

(a) There is a history of recent breast cancer.
(b) The lesion has destroyed the cortex and is not well defined.
(c) The appearances are of a clear isolated defect with a distinct zone of transition.
(d) There is periosteal elevation, Codman's triangle and sunray spicules.
(e) Onion skinning is present.

18. Metastatic bone deposits are:

(a) Commonly from a liver primary.
(b) Embolic through the venous system.
(c) Lytic if from a prostate primary.
(d) Usually located centrally in the skeleton.
(e) Associated with a fracture risk.

19. Dislocation of the shoulder:

(a) Is usually posterior.
(b) If anterior will usually heal and not re-dislocate.
(c) Is usually caused by forced internal rotation.
(d) Can be reduced in the A&E department.
(e) May cause neurological deficit.

20. Patellar dislocation:

(a) Is prevented by a large lateral femoral condyle.
(b) May cause an osteochondral fracture.
(c) If recurrent may require surgical realignment.
(d) Usually occurs medially.
(e) Is treated with early surgical repair.

21. Ankle sprains:

(a) Are very common.
(b) Damage the deltoid ligament.
(c) Should be treated with a plaster cast for 6 weeks.
(d) Are diagnosed on X-ray.
(e) Often result in chronic instability.

22. Symptoms suggestive of nerve root compression include:

(a) Back pain worse on movement.
(b) Pain shooting down the leg into the foot.
(c) Bladder or bowel dysfunction if the cauda equina is involved.
(d) Tingling and numbness in the foot.
(e) Complete loss of power and sensation in the lower limbs (flaccid paralysis).

23. Regarding postoperative complications:

(a) They only occur in unfit old patients.
(b) Fat embolus can cause confusion.
(c) They can be reduced with preoperative antibiotics.
(d) They are minimized by early mobilization.
(e) Deep vein thrombosis (DVT) tends to occur in the first 24 hours after surgery.

24. Concerning fractures:

(a) Those of the radius have a high incidence of avascular necrosis.
(b) They are termed pathological if through abnormal bone.
(c) Open fractures should be treated with plaster immobilization and antibiotics.
(d) Displaced intracapsular hip fractures in the elderly are treated with open reduction and internal fixation (ORIF).
(e) Those of the wrist are usually displaced in a volar (palmar) direction.

25. Children with Perthes disease:

(a) Often present with knee pain.
(b) Are usually teenage girls.
(c) Are more commonly from lower socioeconomic groups.
(d) Have avascular necrosis of the femoral head.
(e) Often have diminished hip abduction.

26. Developmental dysplasia of the hip (DDH):

(a) Can present late with a limp.
(b) Is diagnosed clinically by performing Barlow's and Ortolani's tests.
(c) Is more common in Afro-Caribbean races.
(d) Results in a shallow poorly developed acetabulum.
(e) Is more common in patients with a family history.

27. Slipped upper femoral epiphysis:

(a) Presents with pain radiating down the back of the leg and into the foot.
(b) Usually occurs in infants.
(c) Occurs through the physis.
(d) Is a very common cause of pain and limp in children.
(e) Can present over a long period.

28. A prolapsed intervertebral disc:

(a) Most commonly causes compression of the L4 nerve root.
(b) Produces symptoms that are worse on sitting.
(c) Usually settles without needing surgery.
(d) Is common in the elderly.
(e) Occurs through a weakness in the annulus fibrosis.

29. Scoliosis:

(a) May be secondary to neurological conditions.
(b) Causes a rib hump deformity.
(c) Usually needs surgical correction.
(d) If severe can cause reduced lung volume.
(e) Surgery is relatively simple with no significant risks to the patient.

30. Back pain:

(a) Is a very common condition affecting over half of the population at some time in their lives.
(b) Is always due to disc prolapse.
(c) Can be a presentation of malignancy.
(d) In young patients does not need investigation.
(e) Is treated with prolonged bed rest.

31. Deep vein thrombosis (DVT):

(a) Is a common complication after orthopaedic surgery
(b) Risk can be reduced with mechanical (graduated compression stockings) and chemical (e.g. aspirin or heparin) measures.
(c) May be fatal if pulmonary embolus results.
(d) Is treated with warfarin.
(e) Can result in long-term swelling and pain in the limb.

32. Magnetic resonance imaging (MRI):

(a) Is a safe but expensive investigation for all patients.
(b) Produces images by relaxation of electrons within a magnetic field.
(c) Is particularly useful when looking for meniscal or ligamentous injuries to the knee.
(d) Is more sensitive than plain X-rays for detecting metastases.
(e) Can be used to detect occult fractures.

33. Regarding joint replacements:

(a) They are carried out to relieve pain and improve function of an arthritic joint.
(b) Those of the hip can dislocate if the patient is not careful getting up from a chair.
(c) They are at risk of infection unless strict asepsis is routine in theatre.
(d) The most common cause of failure is loosening.
(e) They are generally successful 90–95% of the time.

34. Ganglions:

(a) If aspirated contain jelly-like fluid.
(b) Are commonly found around the wrist.
(c) May spontaneously disappear.
(d) Never recur following surgery.
(e) May be asymptomatic and left alone.

35. Easily palpable features when examining the knee include:

(a) Menisci.
(b) Anterior cruciate ligament (ACL).
(c) Lateral collateral ligament (LCL).
(d) Posterior cruciate ligament (PCL).
(e) Patellar ligament.

36. Pain in the foot can be due to:

(a) Prolapsed intervertebral disc.
(b) Morton's neuroma.
(c) Hallux valgus.
(d) Stress fracture.
(e) Gout.

37. Clinical features of early primary osteoarthritis include:

(a) Deformity.
(b) Instability.
(c) Swelling.
(d) Muscle wasting.
(e) Effusion.

38. An isotope bone scan:

(a) Is a useful screening test looking for metastases.
(b) Is a specific test but not a sensitive one.
(c) Is performed in three phases.
(d) Requires a small dose of radioactive tracer.
(e) Shows increased uptake in the growth plates of children.

39. Methods of preventing osteoporotic fractures include:

(a) Calcium and vitamin D supplements.
(b) Glucosamine tablets.
(c) Hip protectors.
(d) Bisphosphonates.
(e) Falls clinics.

40. Concerning proximal femoral fractures:

(a) Extracapsular fractures are treated with hip hemiarthroplasty.
(b) The mortality rate is 80% in the year after hip fracture.
(c) Undisplaced intracapsular hip fractures can be treated with operative fixation.
(d) Patients having one hip fracture are at increased risk of a second.
(e) Subtrochanteric fractures are often pathological.

41. The following are operations used for patients with rheumatoid arthritis:

(a) Synovectomy.
(b) Ankle replacement.
(c) High tibial osteotomy.
(d) Shoulder replacement.
(e) Triple fusion.

42. When assessing a patient preoperatively:

(a) It is important to inspect the skin over the operation site.
(b) Heart murmurs should be investigated.
(c) A haemoglobin should be checked on all patients.
(d) For joint replacement it is important to test the urine.
(e) Distal pulses should be palpable.

43. Concerning primary bone tumours:

(a) An osteosarcoma is a benign slow-growing tumour.
(b) Enchondromas are often found in the hand.
(c) A Ewing's tumour is a rare but highly malignant tumour.
(d) Patients present with a painful swelling.
(e) Treatment of malignant lesions includes chemotherapy and surgery.

44. Immediate postoperative care includes:

(a) Elevation of the operated limb.
(b) Analgesia.
(c) Sedation.
(d) Distal and general observations.
(e) Pulse oximetry to measure P_{O_2}.

45. Concerning gait patterns:

(a) High-stepping gait is due to peroneal nerve palsy.
(b) Trendelenburg gait is due to failure of hip adductors.
(c) An antalgic gait is due to pain.
(d) A Trendelenburg gait may be present after total hip replacement.
(e) A short-leg gait is characterized by dipping of the opposite shoulder.

46. Causes of postoperative shortness of breath include:

(a) Atelectasis
(b) Deep vein thrombosis (DVT).
(c) Fluid overload.
(d) Renal failure.
(e) Shock.

47. Special examination tests in orthopaedics include:

(a) The pivot shift for posterior cruciate ligament (PCL) instability.
(b) Thomas' test for fixed flexion of the hip.
(c) Trendelenburg test for hip abductor function.
(d) Sciatic stretch test for nerve root irritation.
(e) Lachman's test for anterior cruciate ligament (ACL) deficiency.

48. Normal variants in a child's development include:

(a) Genu varum.
(b) Genu valgum.
(c) Cubitus varus.
(d) Developmental dysplasia of the hip (DDH).
(e) Rigid flat foot.

49. Causes of a painful joint include:

(a) Rheumatoid arthritis.
(b) Pseudogout.
(c) Tuberculosis.
(d) Avascular necrosis.
(e) Tarsal tunnel syndrome.

50. Causes of swellings around the knee include:

(a) Baker's cyst.
(b) Olecranon bursitis.
(c) Meniscal cyst.
(d) Osteochondroma.
(e) Osteosarcoma.

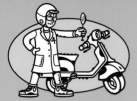
Rheumatology

1. List five causes of anaemia in rheumatoid arthritis (RA).

2. A 23-year-old man consults you with a 2- to 3-year history of gradually worsening lower back pain. The pain is worse first thing in the morning and he feels very stiff for the first 1–2 hours. This stiffness often returns if he sits for long periods. The patient has found that swimming and non-steroidal anti-inflammatory drugs (NSAIDs) help his symptoms. Based on the history, what is the most likely diagnosis, what investigations would you recommend and what results would you expect?

3. What clinical signs might you see in the hands of a patient with limited systemic sclerosis?

4. What is rheumatoid factor?

5. List three factors capable of triggering a flare of systemic lupus erythematosus (SLE).

6. A paediatric rheumatologist sees a 3-year-old girl with a 4-month history of joint pain and swelling. On examination, she is limping and has synovitis of both ankles and her right knee. The child's family doctor has enclosed the results of some blood tests, which show her to have a positive antinuclear antibody (ANA) and raised erythrocyte sedimentation rate (ESR). The rheumatologist makes a diagnosis of juvenile idiopathic arthritis (JIA) and initiates appropriate treatment. What other specialist in the hospital should the rheumatologist refer the patient to and why?

7. What are the main clinical features of antiphospholipid antibody syndrome?

8. A 70-year-old woman consults you complaining of a headache. She rarely suffers with headaches and is concerned, because this one started a week ago and is worsening. What features of the history would point towards a diagnosis of giant cell arteritis?

9. What triad of clinical features is described by Reiter's syndrome?

10. Describe the gait of a patient with a common peroneal nerve injury. At what site is the nerve most vulnerable to injury?

Orthopaedics

1. How can postoperative complications be classified? What systems can be affected by complications?

2. Why do elderly people fall? What are the three typical osteoporotic fractures?

3. Describe the pathology of osteoporosis and list the risk factors.

4. What are the X-ray features of osteoarthritis and what treatment options are available?

5. What features might be present in the history and on examination of a patient with a rupture of the anterior cruciate ligament?

6. What features of an X-ray lesion would make you suspicious of malignancy? List malignant diseases that can present in such a way?

7. How do you differentiate between patients with musculoskeletal back pain and those with a prolapsed intervertebral disc?

8. What is the most important investigation when assessing a patient with an acutely hot swollen joint? Why? List a differential diagnosis.

9. Outline the pathology in haematogenous osteomyelitis.

10. What conditions should be considered when examining a child with a limp and at what age do they present?

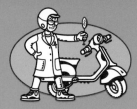

Extended Matching Questions (EMQs)

Rheumatology

1.

(a) Osteoarthritis
(b) Carpal tunnel syndrome
(c) Gout
(d) Trigger finger
(e) Dupuytren's contracture
(f) Ulnar nerve palsy
(g) Pyrophosphate arthropathy
(h) Complex regional pain syndrome
(i) De Quervain's tenosynovitis
(j) Radial nerve palsy
(k) Psoriatic arthropathy

Instruction: *You are examining the right hand of the patients below. Look at the description of the clinical findings and choose the most appropriate diagnosis from the list above.*

1. The muscles of the hypothenar eminence are wasted. Abduction and adduction of the fingers is weak. Sensation over the little finger is reduced.

2. There is pitting of the fingernails. On palpation of the distal interphalangeal (DIP) joints of the middle and ring fingers, there is tender, boggy swelling. The whole length of the index finger is swollen and tender.

3. There is mild generalized swelling of the hand. The skin is pale, cool and extremely hypersensitive, to the extent that light touch produces severe pain. The radial and ulnar pulses are easily palpable.

4. When the patient opens his fist to extend his fingers, the middle finger responds more slowly than the others. In order to fully straighten the digit, the patient has to pull it with his other hand. The palm at the base of the finger feels lumpy.

5. There is bony swelling of all the DIP joints and the base of the thumb. Crepitus can be felt on movements of the thumb.

2.

(a) Serum urate level
(b) Temporal artery biopsy
(c) Measurement of lupus anticoagulant and anticardiolipin antibodies
(d) Synovial fluid aspiration, Gram stain and culture
(e) Nerve conduction studies and electromyography
(f) Erythrocyte sedimentation rate (ESR)
(g) Full blood count
(h) Plain X-ray of the hand and wrist
(i) Thyroid function test
(j) Plain X-ray of the knee

Instruction: *What single investigation from the above list would be the most useful when trying to make a diagnosis in the following situations?*

1. A 63-year-old woman, who is taking low-dose oral corticosteroids and methotrexate for her rheumatoid arthritis, develops swelling and severe pain in her wrist. She is febrile with a temperature of 38.2° and feels generally unwell.

2. A 28-year-old woman is admitted to hospital as an emergency with pleuritic chest pain. She is proven to have a pulmonary embolus and treated accordingly. She has no obvious risk factors for venous thromboembolism. Her past medical history includes recurrent migraines and three previous miscarriages.

3. A 72-year-old man presents with a headache and pain in his jaw when chewing food. He has noticed that the right side of his scalp is tender when he combs his hair.

4. A 36-year-old diabetic man complains of pain and tingling in his left thumb, index and middle fingers. This seems to be worse at night and stops him sleeping.

5. A 65-year-old man who has had one previous attack of gout develops severe pain in his knee. On examination, the joint is hot, swollen and tender. The patient is reluctant to weight bear.

3.

(a) Rheumatoid arthritis
(b) Systemic sclerosis
(c) Systemic lupus erythematosus
(d) Polymyositis
(e) Polymyalgia rheumatica
(f) Kawasaki's disease
(g) Primary Sjögren's syndrome
(h) Takayasu's arteritis
(i) Giant cell arteritis
(j) Wegener's granulomatosis

Instruction: *Read the clinical details of each patient below and decide which is the most appropriate diagnosis from the list above.*

1. A 3-year-old boy develops an acute febrile illness. On examination, he is obviously unwell and has marked cervical lymphadenopathy, an oligoarthritis and desquamation of the skin of his hands and feet.

2. A 44-year-old woman complains that her hands have become slightly swollen and feel tight and itchy. She also finds that her fingers become blue and painful in the cold weather. Apart from heartburn, for which she takes regular antacids, she was previously fit and well. The first thing that her family doctor notices when she walks into his consulting room, is that she has a few telangiectasia on her face.

3. A 48-year-old man becomes acutely breathless and is admitted to hospital as an emergency. He deteriorates rapidly and is intubated and transferred to the intensive care unit for ventilation. A chest X-ray shows multiple shadows in both lung fields, consistent with severe infection or pulmonary haemorrhage. The patient's wife explains to the on-call doctor that he has been unwell for several months with symptoms of joint pain and intermittent skin rashes. He is under regular follow-up with an ear, nose and throat specialist because of recurrent epistaxis.

4. A 56-year-old woman consults her doctor with a 3-month history of weakness of her limbs. She is finding it increasingly difficult to climb the stairs and can no longer carry heavy bags of shopping. She has no pain, but feels very lethargic. Neurological examination of her limbs reveals normal tone and muscle bulk with no fasciculation. Proximal power is reduced at 3/5 in all four limbs. All reflexes are present and normal. Her plantar responses are flexor. Sensory examination is normal.

5. A 45-year-old woman is concerned because her eyes feel dry and gritty and are often red. Her mouth is also dry and she has to take frequent sips of water with her meals. Apart from occasional joint pain, she is otherwise well and has no significant past medical history. Her doctor organizes some blood tests, which reveal a mild normocytic anaemia with a slightly elevated ESR. An autoantibody profile shows the presence of anti-Ro and anti-La antibodies.

4.

(a) Rotator cuff tendinitis
(b) Capsulitis
(c) Osteoarthritis
(d) Polymyalgia rheumatica
(e) Gout
(f) Ruptured long head of biceps
(g) Pancoast tumour
(h) Acute myocardial infarction
(i) Rheumatoid arthritis
(j) Bicipital tendinitis

Instruction: Read the clinical details of each patient below and decide which is the most appropriate diagnosis from the list above.

1. A 31-year-old woman presents with a 2-month history of left shoulder pain, which is gradually worsening. The pain is in the region of her deltoid muscle and is exacerbated by arm movements and lying on her left side. She is now struggling to reach behind her back to fasten her bra strap. On examination, the shoulder looks normal and has a full range of passive movement. However, active movements are painful, and the patient has a painful arc on abduction.

2. A 65-year-old diabetic man develops acute severe pain in his left shoulder whilst walking home from the pub. His wife is worried because he looks grey and sweaty and is slightly short of breath. He seems able to move his arm normally.

3. A doctor is called to a nursing home to visit an elderly woman with advanced dementia. The staff are concerned because they have noticed a swelling in her upper arm. On examination, the swelling is more obvious when the patient flexes her elbow. It feels soft on palpation and does not appear to be tender.

4. A 73-year-old woman presents with a 4-day history of pain in both shoulders. Her arms feel weak and extremely stiff. She has also had some pain in her thighs. The patient's doctor arranges some blood tests, which show that she has a normal full blood count and a very high erythrocyte sedimentation rate (ESR).

5. A 58-year-old man who suffers with chronic obstructive pulmonary disease is admitted to hospital for investigations. Over the past few weeks, he has developed severe pain in his right shoulder and upper arm. The pain is continuous, day and night, and has not responded to any analgesia. The patient complains that he has been losing weight, is more breathless than usual and has coughed up a small amount of blood.

5.

(a) Anti-dsDNA
(b) c-ANCA
(c) p-ANCA
(d) Anti-Sm
(e) Anticentromere
(f) Antigliadin
(g) Anticardiolipin
(h) Anti-Jo1
(i) Antihistone

Instruction: For each of the following patients, select the most characteristic autoantibody profile from the list above.

1. A 59-year-old woman presents with symptoms of Raynaud's phenomenon and dysphagia. On examination, she has painful lesions on her fingers and facial telangiectasia.

2. A 23-year-old man consults his doctor complaining of joint pains, mouth ulcers, lethargy and a rash. His only past medical history is of severe acne, for which he takes minocycline.

3. A 60-year-old man develops acute renal failure. He has been unwell for some time with symptoms of joint pain, skin rashes and several episodes of haemoptysis. On examination, he has a saddle nose deformity.

4. A 45-year-old man presents with abdominal pain, weight loss and a skin rash. On examination, he has wasting of the small muscles of his hands and a purpuric rash on his legs.

5. A 30-year-old woman is admitted to hospital as an emergency with a left hemiparesis. She has a history of recurrent severe migraines, but does not have a headache at present. The doctor examining her notices the rash of livedo reticularis on her lower limbs.

6.

(a) Perthes disease
(b) Juvenile idiopathic arthritis
(c) Developmental dysplasia of the hip
(d) Congenital talipes equinovarus
(e) Slipped upper femoral epiphysis
(f) Septic arthritis
(g) Osteomyelitis
(h) Reactive arthritis
(i) Ewing's tumour.
(j) Osgood–Schlatter disease

Instruction: *Read the clinical details of each patient below and decide which is the most appropriate diagnosis from the list above.*

1. A 13-month-old baby presents with a limp as the child begins to walk. The left leg looks short when compared with the right. The child has a waddling gait but is not in obvious discomfort.

2. A 13-year-old boy presents with a 1-week history of left leg pain radiating from the groin down the thigh and into the knee. The pain is worse on activity and partially relieved by rest. Clinically he has an externally rotated left leg with pain on all movements. The AP X-ray of the hip shows a smaller epiphysis than on the right. The frog lateral view clinches the diagnosis.

3. A 12-year-old boy has been unwell for a few months with pain and swelling in his right knee. He has also been more tired than usual and not himself. On further questioning it becomes clear that other joints are involved. The right knee is swollen with a small effusion. At presentation he is noted to have decreased visual acuity in his right eye.

4. A 14-year-old boy is a keen footballer and presents with bilateral knee pain worse on movement and very tender if touched. On examination he is well and has tenderness over the tibial tubercle just beneath the patellar ligament.

5. A 7-year-old boy presents with a 1-year history of right knee pain gradually increasing. He has a pronounced limp and has been off school for 1 month. On examination the right knee is normal but the hip is irritable and abduction is markedly decreased. X-rays show sclerosis of the femoral head.

6. An 8-week-old baby girl is very ill on the paediatric intensive care unit. She has features of sepsis including a raised temperature and white cell count (WCC), and blood cultures have grown *Staphylococcus aureus*. There is no obvious focus of infection. An ultrasound scan of both hips is normal.

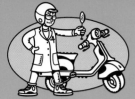
Rheumatology

1. A 60-year-old man consults you with an acute attack of gout affecting his first metatarsophalangeal (MTP) joint. He has had many similar attacks in the past. His past medical history includes hypertension, for which he is taking a thiazide diuretic. He is also taking a non-steroidal anti-inflammatory drug (NSAID). On examination, he is obese with a blood pressure of 180/95. He has tophi in the helices of his ears and in several fingers. His great toe is warm, red, swollen and tender.
   - How would you manage this man?

2. A 75-year-old woman presents to you with a 3-day history of severe headache and left-sided scalp tenderness. She feels generally unwell and has had jaw pain when chewing her food.
   - What would your immediate plans be for investigation and management?

3. A 31-year-old electrician presents with a 4-month history of pain in the small joints of his hands and feet. He finds it difficult to dress himself in the morning because of joint stiffness and is struggling to continue his work. On examination, he has symmetrical synovitis affecting both wrists and most of his metacarpophalangeal (MCP), proximal interphalangeal (PIP) and metatarsophalangeal (MTP) joints. You suspect that he might have rheumatoid arthritis.
   - What investigations should you organize?
   - How will you manage him?

4. A 43-year-old woman consults you with widespread joint pain. She has not been sleeping well at night and is also suffering from fatigue and headaches. Her only significant past medical history is of irritable bowel syndrome. She has had a stressful time recently; her 19-year-old son is an intravenous drug user and has been stealing from her. On examination, her joints have a full range of movement and you can detect no synovitis. However, she has several areas of muscular tenderness over her upper and lower body.
   - What is the most likely diagnosis here?
   - How would you manage her symptoms?

5. A 19-year-old student presents with a 6-month history of intermittent joint pain and aching muscles. She feels very lethargic and has lost a little weight. On systemic enquiry, you discover that she is troubled by mouth ulcers and poor circulation; her fingers become blue and painful during cold weather. The only past medical history of note was an attack of pleurisy 2 years ago. Whilst you are talking to the student, you notice she has an erythematous rash over her nose and cheeks.
   - What is the most likely diagnosis?
   - What investigations should you request?
   - How will you manage the patient's symptoms?

Orthopaedics

1. A 58-year-old insulin-dependent diabetic man presents with osteomyelitis of his left foot. The surgeons are planning to take him to theatre for debridement the next day.
   - What preoperative tests are needed?
   - What measures need to be taken to control his diabetes over the perioperative period?

2. An 80-year-old woman presents with left groin pain after a fall. The leg is short and externally rotated.
   - What is the diagnosis?
   - What is the underlying cause?
   - How would you treat the patient to reduce the risk of further such occurrences?

3. A 40-year-old man presents to casualty with a hot swollen right knee joint. He feels unwell and is barely able to move the knee.
   - What is the differential diagnosis?
   - What is the most important test to perform and why?
   - What is the treatment for this condition?

4. A 9-year-old boy presents with a limp due to pain in his right thigh and knee. The pain started the previous day and he has been unwell with 'flu-like' symptoms for the last few days. On examination, he is apyrexial, well and has a mildly reduced range of movement of his right hip.
- What hip diseases typically present at this age?
- The patient probably has transient synovitis secondary to an upper respiratory tract infection (URTI) but what features on examination suggest it is not a septic arthritis.
- Despite this you want to perform some investigations to exclude infection. Which tests would you perform?

5. A 35-year-old woman presents with a swelling on the dorsum of the wrist, which she has had for several months. It comes and goes but is occasionally painful. On examination there is a firm swelling deep to the skin that is attached to the deep structures. Aspiration obtains clear jelly-like fluid.
- What is the likely diagnosis?
- What feature in the history reassures you that this is a benign lesion?
- Patients very commonly present with swellings and the vast majority are benign. What features would make you worry you had found a rare malignant lesion like a sarcoma?

Rheumatology

1. (a) T—Several subtypes of HLA-DR4 are associated with susceptibility to RA.
(b) F—The hands are commonly involved in RA.
(c) T—The male:female ratio is approximately 1:3.
(d) F—RA is a multisystem disorder.
(e) F—10–30% of RA patients do not carry rheumatoid factor antibodies.

2. (a) F—Obesity is associated with gout.
(b) T—Urate deposition in the renal interstitium and collecting tubules can cause a nephropathy. Urate stones can cause urinary tract obstruction.
(c) F—Radiological changes develop after several years of recurrent gouty attacks.
(d) F—Low-dose salicylate therapy reduces the renal excretion of uric acid and predisposes to gout.
(e) T—This is the commonest joint to be affected by acute gout.

3. (a) T—This can complicate severe spinal diseases.
(b) F—Aortic regurgitation can occur.
(c) T—This and other types of peripheral enthesitis are common in AS.
(d) T—This occurs in approximately one-third of patients with AS.
(e) T—This tends to be a late feature of AS.

4. (a) F—It affects approximately 10% of patients with psoriasis.
(b) T—Some people with psoriatic arthritis never develop psoriasis.
(c) F—There is no correlation between the severity of the arthritis and that of the skin disease.
(d) T—This is a common feature of psoriatic arthropathy.
(e) F—Erosions do occur.

5. (a) F—It affects exocrine glands.
(b) T—B-lymphocytes are activated, resulting in an increase in immunoglobulin production.
(c) T—Rheumatoid arthritis, systemic lupus erythematosus, systemic sclerosis and polymyositis are all causes of secondary Sjögren's syndrome.
(d) T—Neurological manifestations include neuropathies, seizures and hemiparesis.
(e) F—Patients are at an increased risk of developing lymphomas compared to the general population.

6. (a) F—The ESR can be normal.
(b) F—It predominantly targets people over the age of 60 years.
(c) T—This is due to ischaemic optic neuritis, caused by arteritis of the posterior ciliary artery and branches of the ophthalmic arteries.
(d) F—The arteritis is patchy and it is possible to obtain a segment of non-inflamed artery on biopsy.
(e) T—Approximately 50% of patients with GCA have symptoms of PMR.

7. (a) F—It is much more common in women.
(b) F—The joints are normal in fibromyalgia.
(c) T—Approximately 20% of patients with fibromyalgia suffer with anxiety or depression.
(d) T—Patients usually have multiple areas of soft tissue tenderness over the upper and lower body.
(e) F—Cognitive behavioural therapy is not a cure for fibromyalgia, but it can help patients to cope with their symptoms.

8. (a) T—The antibiotic minocycline can trigger drug-induced lupus.
(b) F—The arthritis of SLE is non-erosive.
(c) F—Antinuclear antibodies are detected in more than 95% of patients with SLE.
(d) F—The ESR usually rises during any flare of SLE. The C-reactive protein tends to remain normal unless infection, serositis or synovitis is present.
(e) T—SLE can involve the nervous system, causing seizures, headaches, neuropathies or psychiatric problems.

9. (a) T—It can affect children as well as adults.
(b) F—It causes a proximal myopathy.
(c) T—Up to 15% of adults with inflammatory muscle disease have an underlying malignancy. The association is thought to be much stronger for dermatomyositis than for polymyositis.
(d) T—Scaly, erythematous, papules or plaques called Gottron's papules may develop over the metacarpophalangeal (MCP) and proximal interphalangeal (PIP) joints.
(e) T—This enzyme is released from damaged muscle and is usually at least 10 times the upper limit of normal in active myositis.

10. (a) F—It may be precipitated by overuse of the elbow in any way and is sometimes idiopathic.
(b) F—Pain and tenderness are over the lateral epicondyle at the origin of the forearm extensors.
(c) F—Wrist extension against resistance exacerbates the pain.
(d) T—Enthesitis at any site may be seen, in addition to axial and peripheral joint disease.
(e) T—Symptoms may resolve after rest and avoidance of any precipitating causes.

11. (a) T—The median nerve becomes compressed as it passes through the carpal tunnel at the wrist.
    (b) F—Pain is felt in the thumb, index and middle fingers and the radial half of the ring finger.
    (c) T—Weakness and wasting of the thenar muscles may be seen in advanced cases.
    (d) T—Several endocrine diseases can predispose to carpal tunnel syndrome, including diabetes mellitus, hypothyroidism and acromegaly.
    (e) T—Patients with wrist synovitis are particularly prone to carpal tunnel syndrome.

12. (a) F— They are slow-acting drugs.
    (b) F—They are started soon after diagnosis with the aim of controlling disease activity and delaying the progression of erosive joint damage.
    (c) F—Corticosteroids are often used to suppress disease activity in patients who have not yet responded to their disease-modifying therapy.
    (d) T—Some DMARDs are immunosuppressants.
    (e) T—Most DMARDs have the potential to cause bone marrow suppression.

13. (a) T—Inflammatory joint pain tends to be worse in the morning and improve as the day progresses.
    (b) T—Stiffness that is worse first thing in the morning or after periods of rest is typical of inflammatory arthritis.
    (c) T—Patients with inflammatory arthritis often suffer with constitutional symptoms such as fatigue, fever and weight loss.
    (d) T—Inflammatory arthritis causes 'boggy' joint swelling in contrast to the hard, bony swelling of osteoarthritis.
    (e) T—The increased blood flow to inflamed joints often produces erythema and warmth of the overlying skin.

14. (a) T—It is the rate at which erythrocytes aggregate.
    (b) F—The CRP responds to inflammation faster than the ESR.
    (c) T—The upper limit of normal for the ESR increases with age.
    (d) F—Some patients with definite joint inflammation have a normal ESR.
    (e) T

15. (a) T—This is due to erosive damage.
    (b) F—Periarticular osteoporosis is one of the earliest radiological signs.
    (c) T—Sacroiliitis is found in up to 30% of cases and is usually asymmetrical.
    (d) T—Chondrocalcinosis may also be seen in the triangular cartilage of the wrist.
    (e) T—Early erosions can also be detected using ultrasound.

16. (a) F—It is an aseptic arthritis that develops after a distant infection.
    (b) T—Infections of the gastrointestinal tract are also common triggers.
    (c) F—It is usually an asymmetrical arthritis.
    (d) F—Dactylitis is common.
    (e) T—Symptoms can last for months and relapses are common.

17. (a) F—They are seen in osteoarthritis.
    (b) F—Patients usually develop ulnar deviation at the metacarpophalangeal (MCP) joints and radial deviation at the wrist.
    (c) F—It refers to the hand deformities seen in systemic lupus erythematosus, which result from tenosynovitis rather than erosive damage.
    (d) F—It describes the loss of lumbar lordosis and kyphosis of the thoracic and cervical spines.
    (e) T—Reabsorption of bone at the metacarpals and phalanges causes telescoping of the digits.

18. (a) T—This is a sterile pustular rash on the palms of the hands and soles of the feet.
    (b) F—This rash is a feature of systemic lupus erythematosus.
    (c) T—These are all manifestations of cutaneous vasculitis.
    (d) F—This heliotrope rash is a feature of dermatomyositis. Polymyositis does not affect the skin.
    (e) T—They are often seen on the hands and face of patients with limited systemic sclerosis.

19. (a) T—A positive family history is a risk factor for developing Dupuytren's contracture.
    (b) T—This results in flexion of the fingers.
    (c) F—The ulnar side of the hand is most commonly affected.
    (d) T—Cirrhosis of the liver is a risk factor for Dupuytren's contracture.
    (e) T—There is a risk of recurrence after partial fasciectomy.

20. (a) T—This is due to arterial thrombosis.
    (b) T—Migraines are common.
    (c) F—They should avoid oral contraceptives, which increase thrombotic risk.
    (d) F—Warfarin is teratogenic. Subcutaneous heparin should be used instead.
    (e) T

21. (a) F—Synovial fluid has a cloudy appearance if the cell count is high. This can be due to septic arthritis or joint inflammation. Infection should always be excluded.
    (b) F—The absence of organisms on microscopy does not exclude infection. Gram stain and culture should be performed.
    (c) T—Polarized light is required to examine the birefringence of crystals.
    (d) T
    (e) F—They show weak positive birefringence.

22. (a) T—Pain is felt in between the metatarsal heads and often radiates along the adjacent borders of the two affected toes.
(b) F—This causes pain in the region of the Achilles tendon.
(c) T—Pain is felt in the great toe.
(d) T—This commonly affects the first metatarsophalangeal (MTP) joint.
(e) T—This can, but does not always, cause forefoot pain.

23. (a) T—It can be a consequence of bone marrow suppression.
(b) T—This is due to autoimmune destruction of platelets.
(c) T—Active inflammation due to any cause can cause a reactive thrombocytosis.
(d) T—As above.
(e) F—It causes thrombocytopenia.

24. (a) T—Any prolonged, severe illness in childhood can delay growth.
(b) T
(c) F—It affects between one and four joints.
(d) F—They are often HLA-B27 positive.
(e) F—It is associated with an increased risk of uveitis.

25. (a) F—Women are affected more commonly than men.
(b) T—This can be severe and lead to ischaemic changes of the digits.
(c) F—Pulmonary or renal involvement is most likely to be fatal.
(d) T—This can be primary or secondary to pulmonary fibrosis.
(e) T—The pericardium can also be affected.

26. (a) F—High doses of corticosteroids are usually required initially and treatment often has to be continued for months or years.
(b) T
(c) T
(d) F—The small vessel vasculitides (such as Wegener's granulomatosis and microscopic polyangiitis) cause significant morbidity and mortality.
(e) T

27. (a) T—This can cause a symmetrical peripheral neuropathy, with a 'glove and stocking' distribution.
(b) F
(c) T—This results from posterior tibial nerve compression.
(d) T—This usually affects the borders of adjacent toes.
(e) F

28. (a) T—Fever may be a feature of active SLE and is often present in the absence of infection.
(b) F—This occurs in systemic sclerosis.
(c) T—Patients may develop rashes on light-exposed areas.
(d) F—This is not a recognized feature of SLE.
(e) F—This is not a recognized feature of SLE.

29. (a) F
(b) F
(c) T
(d) T
(e) F

Please see Figure 11.9 (p. 73) for the diseases associated with secondary Sjögren's syndrome.

30. (a) F—They reflect the disease activity of SLE, not RA.
(b) T—Patients with primary Sjögren's syndrome can have very high titres of rheumatoid factor.
(c) T—Although, they are not present in all cases.
(d) T—They are found in 80% of patients with active Wegener's granulomatosis.
(e) F—They are found in 5–10% of the normal population.

31. (a) F
(b) T
(c) T
(d) F
(e) T

Please see Figure 9.11 (p. 55) for the extra-articular features of RA.

32. (a) T
(b) F—It causes splenomegaly.
(c) F—It causes leucopenia rather than a leucocytosis.
(d) T—This is a consequence of leucopenia.
(e) F—Patients are usually rheumatoid factor positive.

33. (a) T
(b) F—They are the cause of pseudogout.
(c) T—They can cause pyrophosphate arthropathy.
(d) T—Haemochromatosis predisposes to pseudogout and pyrophosphate arthropathy.
(e) T—Monosodium urate and calcium pyrophosphate dihydrate can coexist in some joints.

34. (a) F—Pannus is found in rheumatoid arthritis.
(b) T—This is known as the lupus 'band' test.
(c) T—The sural nerve is sometimes biopsied.
(d) T
(e) T—The findings are similar to those of SLE.

35. (a) T—It is derived from the breakdown of purine bases, which are components of nucleic acids.
(b) F—Approximately two-thirds is renally excreted.
(c) F—Levels are higher in males than in females from puberty until the menopause.
(d) F—It is usually due to reduced uric acid breakdown.
(e) T—This causes a massive increase in cell breakdown and, therefore, uric acid synthesis.

36. (a) T
(b) T
(c) T
(d) T
(e) F

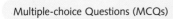

37. (a) F—It presents most commonly in middle-aged men.
(b) T—Microaneurysms are commonly found in the renal arteries and the coeliac axis.
(c) T—Polyarteritis nodosa commonly affects the peripheral nerves.
(d) F—There is an association with hepatitis B antigenaemia.
(e) T

38. (a) T
(b) T   All these conditions can result from overuse.
(c) T
(d) F
(e) F

39. (a) T
(b) T
(c) T   Fever and rashes are also common symptoms.
(d) T
(e) T

40. (a) F—Hypothyroidism may be associated with CPPD deposition.
(b) F—Hyperparathyroidism may be associated with CPPD deposition.
(c) T—See Figure 13.8 (p. 96) for other predisposing diseases.
(d) F
(e) F

41. (a) T
(b) T
(c) F
(d) T
(e) F

42. (a) F
(b) T
(c) T   Please see Figure 9.12 (p. 56) for the radiological signs of RA.
(d) F
(e) F

43. (a) F—It is not possible to accurately estimate bone mineral density from radiographs. However, they can give an indication of osteopenia.
(b) T—An early menopause results in a longer duration of relative oestrogen deficiency.
(c) T—This is secondary to vertebral wedge compression fractures.
(d) F—It Is defined as bone mineral density of greater than 2.5 standard deviations below the mean.
(e) T

44. (a) T—Vascular shunting of blood through diseased bone may occasionally lead to high output cardiac failure.
(b) T—Bony expansion of the skull can cause compression of the eighth cranial nerve or conductive deafness.
(c) T—This develops in less than 1% of cases.
(d) T—This is a rare complication of vertebral Paget's disease.
(e) T—Secondary osteoarthritis can occur.

45. (a) T
(b) F—These are a feature of osteomalacia.
(c) T
(d) T
(e) T

Orthopaedics

1. (a) F—OA is very common and can normally be managed without surgery.
(b) F—Methotrexate is a disease-modifying drug used in rheumatoid arthritis.
(c) T—Early treatment of OA should include physiotherapy to maintain function.
(d) T—NSAIDs are useful in controlling symptoms of OA.
(e) T—Fusion is commonly performed around the foot and ankle for OA.

2. (a) F—OA is a degenerative arthritis.
(b) T—These are the four classical features of OA on X-ray.
(c) T—Severe lower limb deformities cause abnormal loading of joints and predispose to OA.
(d) T
(e) F—Water content increases in OA and decreases in ageing.

3. (a) F—It is often affected by rheumatoid arthritis.
(b) T—Herberden's nodes occur here.
(c) T
(d) T
(e) T

4. (a) T—Patellar crepitus can be felt (and sometimes heard) when examining an arthritic knee.
(b) T—Walking distance is reduced.
(c) F—Internal rotation in flexion is usually the first movement lost.
(d) F—OA is not a systemic disorder.
(e) T—OA is a degenerative disorder.

5. (a) T—Arthrodesis is often performed around the foot and ankle.
(b) F—This is performed for carpal tunnel syndrome.
(c) T—Replacement is now routine for the hip, knee, shoulder and elbow.
(d) F—This procedure is for fractures.
(e) T—Osteotomy is usually performed around the knee to correct a deformity and redistribute load.

6. (a) T—This is due to the use of contaminated needles.
(b) F—These patients are at risk of salmonella osteomyelitis.
(c) F
(d) T—Patients with chronic renal disease have a reduced immune response.
(e) F

7. (a) T—It is often difficult to distinguish between them.
(b) T—Although not common, inflammatory conditions can present with an acutely painful joint.
(c) T—This is the most important diagnosis to exclude.
(d) F—Discitis is an infection in the intervertebral disc.
(e) F—DDH presents with hip pain.

8. (a) F—It can present at any age.
(b) F—It usually occurs following surgery or trauma.
(c) F—In post-surgical osteomyelitis there is usually dead bone present which acts as a nidus for infection and needs to be removed.
(d) F—Osteomyelitis can occur after open fractures.
(e) F—The most common infecting organism is *Staphylococcus aureus.*

9. (a) F—It is becoming more common, partly due to immigration and increasing HIV/AIDS.
(b) T—Spread can occur throughout the body
(c) T
(d) T—This is called vertebra plana.
(e) F—Mycobacteria are notoriously difficult to culture and it may take 6 weeks.

10. (a) T—ACL-deficient knees show abnormal forward movement.
(b) T—The ACL is frequently injured in this way.
(c) F—If completely ruptured, the ACL does not heal.
(d) F—Instability is the main symptom with patient complaining of the knee 'giving way'.
(e) T—Using either the hamstring tendons or patellar ligament (bone–patella–bone).

11. (a) T—Swelling develops quickly.
(b) T—The PCL is another intra-articular ligament.
(c) T—The peripheral rim of the meniscus has a blood supply and therefore bleeding and a haemarthrosis can result.
(d) T—Bleeding occurs after fracture.
(e) T—It may be associated with osteochondral fragments.

12. (a) F—They are more common in the medial meniscus.
(b) T—Large bucket handle tears often cause locking of the knee.
(c) T—Particularly in older patients.
(d) T—Unstable knees predispose to meniscal tears.
(e) F—Some can be repaired but the majority are excised.

13. (a) T
(b) T—Primary osteoporosis is age related.
(c) T—This is the most important cause of osteoporosis.
(d) T—Immobilized patients develop osteoporosis.
(e) T—These are an important cause of secondary osteoporosis, e.g. hyperparathyroidism.

14. (a) F—It is usually due to lack of vitamin D.
(b) T—These are stress fractures that are often seen around the hip or pelvis.
(c) T—Due to lack of mineralization.
(d) F
(e) T—Symptoms resolve with this treatment.

15. (a) T—The patient may present with a fracture.
(b) F—Increased bone turnover, abnormal bony architecture and impending fractures cause pain but most patients do not have pain.
(c) T—They are effective at reducing pain.
(d) T—Bleeding is often significant at surgery.
(e) T—Sabre tibia is classical.

16. (a) T
(b) T—So-called spinal claudication is typical of spinal stenosis.
(c) T
(d) F—The pain tends to be aching and radiates into the leg.
(e) T—It is more common in these patients.

17. (a) T—A history of previous cancer is important.
(b) T—A poorly defined zone of transition is suspicious.
(c) F—These appearances suggest a benign lesion.
(d) T—These are the classic X-ray features of a primary malignant bone tumour.
(e) T—This is another feature associated with malignancy.

18. (a) F—Bone metastases are usually from lung, breast, prostate, kidney or thyroid.
(b) T—Metastases spread to the axial skeleton through a plexus of veins.
(c) F—Prostatic metastases tend to be sclerotic.
(d) T—The spine, pelvis and proximal femur are common sites.
(e) T—A patient may present with a pathological fracture secondary to metastasis.

19. (a) F—Anterior dislocation is much more common.
(b) F—There is a 70–80% chance of re-dislocation in young active patients.
(c) F—The arm is in the overhead position of abduction and external rotation.
(d) T—There are many techniques described and this is a very satisfying procedure for junior doctors to perform.
(e) T—A traction injury can occur to the axillary or musculocutaneous nerve.

44. (a) T—On a Braun's frame or in a Bradford sling.
   (b) T—A comfortable pain-free patient is the goal.
   (c) F—Sedation is not given postoperatively as this will lower the conscious level further.
   (d) T—General: pulse, temperature, and blood pressure. Distal: neurovascular status.
   (e) F—The pulse oximeter measures oxygen saturation not the Po_2.

45. (a) T—This is due to foot drop; the patient must lift the leg high to avoid dragging it on the floor.
   (b) F—It is due to failure of hip abductors.
   (c) T—The patient quickens and shortens the step on the painful limb.
   (d) T—The abductor can be defunctioned.
   (e) F—It is the shoulder on the short side that dips.

46. (a) T—Reduced numbers of functioning alveoli may result in shortness of breath.
   (b) F—Unless the DVT becomes a pulmonary embolism.
   (c) T—Fluid overload can cause pulmonary oedema.
   (d) T—Renal failure may cause a metabolic acidosis, and in response to this the respiratory rate is increased to 'blow off' the excess CO_2.
   (e) T—Shock is an important cause of increased respiratory rate because of inadequate tissue perfusion.

47. (a) F—The pivot shift is a test for ACL deficiency.
   (b) T—By abolishing the lumbar lordosis, the true degree of fixed flexion is observed.
   (c) T—The pelvis tilts towards the unsupported leg.
   (d) T—Commonly L5 or S1.
   (e) T—The tibia moves forward on a fixed femur.

48. (a) T—As infants, children are 'bow legged'.
   (b) T—Later, as children grow, they become more 'knock kneed'.
   (c) F—Normally the elbow is in valgus. A varus carrying angle usually results from a fracture.
   (d) F—This is pathological.
   (e) F—Flexible flat feet are common but a rigid one suggests a pathological cause.

49. (a) T—Patients can present with a single joint arthritis.
   (b) T—This is a common cause of joint pain and swelling.
   (c) T—Tuberculosis can spread to joints.
   (d) T—It usually occurs in the hip but is also found in the knee.
   (e) F—Tarsal tunnel syndrome is a cause of foot pain caused by compression of the posterior tibial nerve.

50. (a) T—The cyst is felt behind the knee and is usually due to degenerative disease.
   (b) F—This bursa is over the tip of the elbow.
   (c) T—Meniscal cysts are more common laterally and are due to meniscal tears that have a valve-like action, allowing synovial fluid to be pumped out.
   (d) T—Osteochondromas are benign tumours that are often found around the knee.
   (e) T—These are very rare tumours but they can occur here.

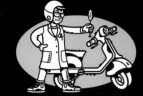

SAQ Answers

Rheumatology

1. • Chronic disease.
   • Autoimmune haemolysis.
   • Felty's syndrome.
   • Iron deficiency secondary to gastrointestinal blood loss from non-steroidal anti-inflammatory drugs (NSAIDs).
   • Bone marrow suppression secondary to disease-modifying antirheumatic drugs (DMARDs).

2. The history is suggestive of ankylosing spondylitis. Plain X-rays of the patient's lumbar spine and pelvis should be requested. There may be sclerosis of the sacroiliac joints and squaring of the vertebral bodies, with or without syndesmophyte formation. A full blood count may reveal a mild anaemia and the erythrocyte sedimentation rate (ESR) and C-reactive protein (CRP) will be raised during active disease.

3. • Sclerodactyly.
   • Telangiectasia.
   • Calcinosis.
   • Ischaemic changes, such as gangrene.

4. Rheumatoid factor is an antibody directed against the Fc fragment of IgG antibody. Rheumatoid factors may be of any immunoglobulin class, although IgM is the rheumatoid factor that is most commonly measured.

5. • Overexposure to sunlight.
   • Oral contraceptive pill.
   • Infection.
   • Stress.

6. An ophthalmologist should examine the child's eyes with a slit-lamp to look for signs of chronic anterior uveitis. She has oligoarticular JIA and a positive ANA, which means she has a significant risk of developing eye disease.

7. • Arterial and venous thrombosis.
   • Recurrent fetal loss.
   • Thrombocytopenia.

8. A history of scalp tenderness, jaw claudication or visual disturbance raises suspicion of giant cell arteritis. Approximately 50% of patients have symptoms of polymyalgia rheumatica, so pain and stiffness in the shoulder and pelvic girdles are also suggestive.

9. Arthritis, urethritis and conjunctivitis.

10. The foot is plantar flexed and inverted ('foot drop'). The patient takes high steps, flicking the foot forwards to avoid tripping over it. The common peroneal nerve is most vulnerable to injury where it winds around the neck of the fibula.

Orthopaedics

1. Any postoperative complications can be:
   • Immediate (within hours).
   • Early (days).
   • Late (months).
   and:
   • Local (i.e. related to that specific operation).
   • General (simply because the patient is having an operation).
   Any system can be affected by postoperative complications:
   • Respiratory: e.g. chest infection.
   • Cardiovascular: e.g. left ventricular failure (LVF) or myocardial infarction (MI).
   • Gastrointestinal (GI): ileus or upper GI bleeding.
   • Genitourinary: urinary retention.
   • Skin: pressure sores.

2. Elderly people fall because of:
   • Intrinsic factors:
     —Acute medical conditions: e.g. cerebrovascular accident (CVA), transient ischaemic attack (TIA), atrial fibrillation (AF).
     —Diminished senses: e.g. poor eyesight
     —Reduced reflexes: ageing produces an inability to recover from a slight stumble increasing falls.
     —Poor mobility: e.g. arthritis or previous CVA.
   • Extrinsic factors:
     —Poor housing
     —Lack of social services.
   When elderly people do fall the three typical osteoporotic fractures are:
   1. Spine.
   2. Wrist.
   3. Hip.

3. Osteoporosis results from an imbalance of osteoblastic and osteoclastic activity. If the osteoclasts remove more bone than is being laid down by the osteoblasts then a net loss of bone results. The bony trabeculae become thinner with a decreased number of connections.
   Risk factors for developing osteoporosis include:
   • Age.
   • Female sex.
   • Family history.
   • Small size.
   • Caucasian race.
   • Early menopause.
   • Smoking.
   • Alcoholism.
   • Lack of weight-bearing activity.

233

5.

1. Anticentromere (e). This patient has limited systemic sclerosis, which is strongly associated with anticentromere antibodies.
2. Antihistone (i). This man has drug-induced systemic lupus erythematosus, as a consequence of his minocycline therapy. Antihistone antibodies are commonly found in this condition.
3. c-ANCA (b). This man has Wegener's granulomatosis. 80% of patients are c-ANCA positive.
4. p-ANCA (c). This patient has polyarteritis nodosa, which is associated with p-ANCA.
5. Anticardiolipin (g). This patient has antiphospholipid antibody syndrome.

Orthopaedics

1.

1. Prostate metastasis (a). The history of urinary dysfunction suggests prostate. Metastases from prostate cancer are sclerotic (the others being lytic).
2. Osteosarcoma (g). Although rare, primary malignant tumours do occur in children and metastases are unheard of in this age group. The level of pain is suspicious but it is the X-ray features that give away the diagnosis.
3. Myeloma (c). The fracture under normal loads should raise suspicion. The X-ray features are typical of myeloma as are the high ESR and skull lesions.
4. Osteochondroma (i). The history is benign, of mild discomfort over long periods, and the X-ray appearance is typical of a benign lesion, in this case an osteochondroma.
5. Breast metastasis (f). I have not told you that she had a breast lump. She has a malignant spinal lesion causing spinal cord compression. The normal investigations exclude all the other potential sources of primary malignancy (except bowel carcinoma, but this rarely metastasizes to the spine) leaving breast carcinoma as the most likely.
6. Lung metastasis (b). The history of smoking and an abnormal chest X-ray give away the diagnosis.

2.

1. Posterior cruciate ligament rupture (i). The history is typical with a backwardly directed force on the tibia. The posterior sag is pathognomonic for PCL rupture.
2. Medial collateral sprain (e). The history suggests medial ligament sprain and the fact that she could bear weight afterwards suggests a less serious injury. Tenderness at the joint line would be the meniscus but above is more likely to be medial collateral. The absence of an effusion excludes an anterior cruciate ligament rupture.
3. Osteoarthritis (c). The history is typical for OA with gradually increasing pain, a varus deformity and crepitus.
4. Anterior cruciate ligament rupture (a). The history of a skiing injury and the patient hearing a pop or feeling something go is typical. The presence of an effusion makes it more likely. Often knees such as these are difficult to examine initially but later will have positive Lachman's and pivot shift tests.
5. Medial meniscal tear (b). The history of twisting injury, things settling but persistent niggling symptoms is typical. Joint line tenderness and an effusion also suggest meniscal injury.
6. Patellar tendon rupture (j). In this case the history is not helpful but examination findings of loss of straight leg raise with swelling and tenderness below the patella give the diagnosis.

3.

1. Paget's disease (a). The abnormal bony architecture and high alkaline phosphatase give the diagnosis.
2. Rickets (c). The history is typical for rickets, as are the clinical and X-ray features.
3. Osteoporosis (d) presenting with vertebral fractures. The history with deformity and X-ray features all point to osteoporotic vertebral fractures. The normal blood tests exclude pathological causes of fractures.
4. Leukaemia (f). The history of prolonged illness with aches and pains suggests a generalized disorder. The low WCC is also suggestive of a haematological disorder and a sterile hip washout makes septic arthritis very unlikely. Leukaemia does occasionally present with musculoskeletal symptoms.
5. Osteogenesis imperfecta (h). The history of 'spontaneous' or low-violence fractures is typical. These cases are often initially diagnosed as non-accidental injury but here the X-ray shows abnormal bone.
6. Osteoid osteoma (i). The history is typical with intense pain relieved by NSAIDs. The X-ray and CT finding are typical.

4.

1. Osteoarthritis (a) of the first MTP joint (hallux rigidus). The pain in the toe-off stage is typical as the patient has lost extension. Walking boots can relieve the pain by minimizing this movement. Clinical features are typical of OA anywhere, with osteophytes (dorsal bump) and crepitus.
2. Reiter's syndrome (c). A syndrome of arthritis, conjunctivitis and urethritis. It is more common in men but does occur in women.
3. Psoriatic arthropathy (i). Commonly affects the hands which can be significantly deformed.
4. Septic arthritis (d). Can be a difficult diagnosis to make in the elderly. Her raised WCC and temperature point to an infective cause.
5. Gout (e). Typical history and the usual joint. The serum uric acid is often normal during an acute episode.
6. Ankylosing spondylitis (g). The condition tends to present in early adult life and the spine is commonly affected and stiffens, eventually ankylosing. The sacroiliac joints are commonly involved.

5.

1. Spinal stenosis (b). The history is typical and pain is often worse on extension. The X-ray often only shows osteoarthritis and a CT or MRI scan will confirm the presence of spinal stenosis.
2. Spinal metastases (f). The history sounds sinister, with unrelenting pain. The X-ray showing loss of the pedicle (winking owl) means bony destruction by tumour.
3. Discitis (d). Often this condition presents late after the patient has had a number of normal investigations. This patient is at risk of sepsis, having diabetes and chronic renal failure. The X-ray shows the typical features of long-standing discitis.
4. Cauda equina syndrome (j). This is a typical history. Bilateral symptoms are suspicious. Any patient with sciatica and new urinary or bowel disturbance should be investigated urgently.
5. Acute low back pain (g). Very common and usually resolves. Note the absence of leg pain.
6. Spondylolisthesis (a). Fast bowlers in cricket are at increased risk. The X-ray features in this case are diagnostic.

6.

1. Developmental dysplasia of the hip (c). Late-presenting DDH presents with a painless limp and leg length discrepancy. All the other conditions on the list will present with pain.
2. Slipped upper femoral epiphysis (e). The patient is the correct age and the history of pain is typical. The femoral head in SUFE rotates posteriorly and leaves an externally rotated leg. The frog lateral X-ray shows the slip more obviously than the AP X-ray.
3. Juvenile idiopathic arthritis (b). Presentation with a monoarthritis is common, with other joints involved later. Generalized symptoms suggest a systemic disorder. The presence of eye symptoms is worrying as blindness can result.
4. Osgood–Schlatter disease (j). The disease is often bilateral and occurs during the adolescent years. Tender swollen tibial tuberosities are present bilaterally.
5. Perthes disease (a). The boy is the right age to have Perthes and the history of knee pain is typical. The loss of abduction is worrying as it could mean impending joint subluxation. The sclerosis of the femoral head is due to avascular necrosis.
6. Osteomyelitis (g). Diagnosis is difficult in the very young child. In this case the child obviously has an infection. In the absence of an obviously swollen joint and with a normal hip ultrasound scan the most likely cause is osteomyelitis.

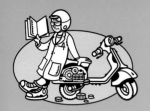

Index